GW00494130

Illustrated Massage
for
Infants and Toddlers

Editors-in-Chief   Qu Jingxi

Wang Qinglin

Translator   Chen Ping

Shandong Science and Technology Press

First Edition 1997
ISBN 7 − 5331 − 2049 − 3

Illustrated Massage for Infants and Toddlers

Editors-in-Chief	Qu Jingxi Wang Qinglin
Deputy Editors	Wang Huanguo Liu Rihe
	Gao Lianjun
Translator	Chen Ping
Illustrations	Liu Huiyu Guo Lei
English Language Editor	Marcia Veach (USA)
Responsible Editors	Li Yu Zhong Pengjun

Published by Shandong Science and Technology Press
16 Yuhan Road, Jinan 250002, China
Printed by Jinan Xinhua Printing House, China
Distributed by China International Book Trading Corporation
35 Chegongzhuang Xilu, Beijing 100044, China
P.O. Box 399, Beijing, China

Printed in the People's Republic of China

Preface

The rapid development of medical science and increased use of medical technology have brought about iatrogenic and drug-induced disorders, which can be mystifying and even alarming. So nonpharmaceutic therapies have become more and more popular.

Massage therapy has a long historical development and is one of the brilliant components of traditional therapies. More and more medical practitioners and health-conscious people focus on massage therapy because of its special procedures, effectiveness and other advantages which other therapies can never replace.

In order to advance Traditional Chinese Medicine (TCM) and develop applications for massage therapy which can prevent and treat diseases, we wrote this illustrated series based on our decades of clinical experience. There are four volumes in this series including *Illustrated Massage for Infants and Toddlers*, *Illustrated Massage for Pregnant Women*, *Illustrated Massage for Couples* and *Illustrated Massage for Middle-Aged and Older Adults*.

This volume is the illustrated introduction to physiological and pathological characteristics in infants and toddlers, and selection and combination of manipulations for treating commonly seen disorders based both on the characteristics and Syndrome Identification. The five chapters include general

1

knowledge, basic manipulations, commonly used sequences, special massage at points and areas on the hand, and the prevention and treatment of commonly encountered disorders. 232 illustrations are included to demonstrate the manipulations discussed in the book and make this therapy easy to understand, learn and master.

CONTENTS

AN OVERVIEW

MANIPULATIONS

COMMONLY USED SEQUENCES

3

TREATMENTS USING
HAND POINTS AND AREAS

4

TREATMENT FOR COMMONLY ENCOUNTERED DISORDERS

ATTACHED FINGERS

AN OVERVIEW

Physiological and Pathological Characteristics

With their Yang and Yin rising, infants are overflowing with vigor. But they have not completely developed, so don't have sufficient Qi and Blood, and their Zang and Fu Organs are immature. They also have weak muscles, tendons, channels and collaterals, and pulse conditions. It is important to fully understand the physiological and pathological characteristics of infants and infant disorders because they are directly related to the therapeutic effects of massage treatments.

Physiological Characteristics

Immature Zangfu Organs with insufficient Qi and Blood In infants, the body type, functions of Zangfu Organs, Qi and Blood, like the growing young shoot of a tree, are not well developed. Many ancient TCM practitioners described this: Though the skin, hair, muscles, tendons, bones, brain, marrow, five Zang Organs, six Fu Organs, nutrition and body resistance, and Qi and Blood have been formed, they are not well developed and strong enough. This is especially true of some important Zang Organs such as the Lung, Spleen and Kidney. The Lung governs Qi; the Spleen functions

3

to transport and transform nutrients to determine the condition of the acquired constitution; and the Kidney dominates bones to determine the condition of the congenital constitution. Invasion of external pathogens, cough, asthma and fever may occur if Lung Qi is insufficient; malnutrition, diarrhea, and loss of appetite come from Deficiency of Spleen Qi if the Spleen is deficient; long-term deficiency-natured disorders, and five kinds of retardation and flaccidity are all closely related to Deficiency of Kidney Qi.

All of these disorders can be prevented or remedied by suitable treatments such as the massage techniques discussed in this book.

Overflowing with vigor and rapid development With the rising of Yang Qi, infants grow and develop rapidly, just like grass growing with vigor. *Qian Jin Yao Fang* (*Thousand Ducat Formulas*) states: "An infant only 60 days after birth can smile in response to something; he can turn his own body over in 100 days when the Ren Channel is developed; he can sit without support in 180 days when the bone system in the lower part of the body is developed; he can lie face down and crawl in 210 days when the bone system in the upper part of the body is developed; he can stand and walk without support in 300 days when the patella and knee joints are developed." These characteristics are due to the function of Pure Yang which refers to the rising Yang during infancy.

Pathological Characteristics

The pathological characteristics in infants are determined by the physiological characteristics. These include:

4

Increased susceptibility to illness The functions of Zangfu and body resistance in infants are too weak to counter the attacks of pathogenic factors, so infants tend to contract diseases more readily. Also, the progress of the illness occurs rapidly, as described by *Wen Bing Tiao Bian* (*Systematic Identification On Febrile Diseases*) : just like lightning.

In infants, the function of the Kidney, Spleen and Lung are often in an insufficient state.

As the Kidney is insufficient, the infant may suffer from five kinds of retardation and flaccidity* . Also, if Deficient Kidney Water fails to nourish Liver Wood leading to Deficiency of Liver Yin, then rising of Liver Wind occurs.

As the Spleen is deficient, the infant may suffer from digestive disorders which are marked by vomiting, diarrhea, food stagnation and abdominal pain.

As the Lung is deficient, the infant may suffer from respiratory disorders which are marked by high fever, cough, asthma and mucus accumulation.

The seriousness of an illness tends to change rapidly With weak body resistance, the infant tends to suffer from invasion of pathogenic factors, an Excess Syndrome. But owing to the weakness of Vital Qi, the Excess Syndrome tends to become a Deficiency Syndrome, or a complex situation in which an Excess becomes complicated by a Deficiency Syndrome. For instance, an Exterior Syndrome caused by invasion of Wind Heat is marked by fever, cough and asthma. After this, coma, convulsion and spasm of limbs will occur if Heart Yang is insufficient, as the invading pathogens can reach the Interior of the body. An Excess Syndrome caused by improper food intake and marked by severe diarrhea can become Yin Deficiency and even Exhaustion Syn-

5

drome if too many Body Fluids are lost.

With pure Zang Qi, recovery is expedited The Heart and Liver are generally sufficient in infants. This is why infants are vigorous, active, and quick in their reactions. Also, pathogenic factors in infants are more simple, so disorders in infants are easier to heal with proper treatment and nursing care as described by *Jing Yue Quan Shu* (*Medical Compendium of Zhang Jingyue*): "With clear Zang Qi, infants have a good reaction to medicine. One dose of decoction, if used properly, can heal sometimes. It's not as difficult as treating an adult."

---

* Note: Five kinds of retardation refer to five kinds of delayed development including retardation in standing, walking, hair growth, tooth eruption and the faculty of speech.

Five kinds of flaccidity refer to five kinds of debility in the neck, the back of the neck, muscles, extremities and mastication.

Mechanism

The TCM Perspective

In TCM theory it is said that a breakdown of the balance between Yin and Yang leads to a relative Excess or Deficiency of Yin or Yang. This causes disorders of Qi and Blood, or Zangfu disharmony. As both the Interior and Exterior of the body are considered to be an organic whole, local points or areas on the surface correspond to the Zangfu. The flow of Qi and Blood through the channels and collaterals connects the Zangfu and four limbs, nine orifices, and five sense organs. Manipulations performed on the Exterior regulate the flow of Qi and Blood circulating in the channels and collaterals, and thus harmonize the functions of the related Zangfu. The strength, angle, depth, speed and direction of manipulation are determined by the medical goal.

The Modern Scientific Perspective

Modern medical research has demonstrated that massage improves skin respiration, and increases skin temperature, brightness and elasticity. After treatment, the circulation of blood and lymph is accelerated. The number of phagocytes (WBC) is significantly increased. Gastrointestinal peristalsis and digestive gland secretion also improve. In addition, most manipulations have an analgesic effect. This therapy improves both general and local metabolism, as well as bioelectrical conductivity, and blood circulation to the heart, brain and kidneys.

Further research using new methods should demonstrate techniques by which energy can be transformed through manipulation and used to stimulate the patient's body to self-regulation and healing.

MANIPULATIONS

Requirements
and Procedures
for Manipulations

The type of manipulation is determined by the physiological and pathological characteristics of infants. Apart from the correct selection of points and areas to be massaged, the appropriate selection of manipulations and their proper application are directly related to therapeutic effect. Basic requirements call for infant and toddler massage to be brisk, gentle, balanced and accurate.

Brisk Manipulations are rapidly done with a light, but penetrating touch, over a short period of time; take care not to damage the child's skin.

Gentle The manipulations are done softly and flexibly.

Balanced The force applied should be moderate—neither too heavy nor too light. The hand movements should be steady, but neither too fast nor too slow.

Accurate The manipulations should be concentrated at the selected point or area using only the force necessary to penetrate deeply.

Any single manipulation's force and duration is determined by the individual situation.

The practitioner should concentrate during manipulating.

Reinforcing and reducing These are discussed within

each chapter and section. In general, they are determined by the direction of manipulation and the amount of force applied.

Contraindications
and Main Points
for Attention

In order to avoid unexpected complications during massage, practitioners should know the contraindications for the use of massage, and some other important points for attention.

Contraindications

1. Acute infectious diseases such as scarlet fever and cerebritis.
2. Unhealed fractures.
3. Skin disorders, burns, scalds, ulcers or sores.
4. Acute internal bleeding, manifested by vomiting or spitting of blood.
5. Overeating or excess hunger.

Main Points for Attention

1. Treatment room should be quiet and warm. Smoking should be absolutely forbidden.
2. Correct diagnosis should be determined before manipulating.
3. The practitioner should keep her hands smooth and fingernails trimmed to avoid damaging an infant's skin

13

while manipulating; watches and bracelets should be removed.

4. In general, manipulations can be performed with both hands, but they are usually done with the left hand.

5. The practitioner should keep his massaging hand warm; manipulations should be done gently and flexibly, gradually increasing the frequency.

6. Media should be selected according to Syndrome Identification.

7. Points in the upper body should be massaged first, then those in the lower body; main points first, then supplementary points.

8. Keep the infant in the room after the massage, particularly those who are still sweating.

Commonly
Used Media

Media are the substances used on the massaged areas.
Proper use of a medium not only protects the skin from
damage during massage, but also improves the therapeutic effects of manipulations. The medium for a massage is chosen according to the constitution of the infant. Warm and hot-natured media are recommended
for a Deficiency Cold-natured constitution; while cold,
cool and bland-natured ones are better for a Heat-na-
tured constitution. There are several commonly used
media.

Warm and Hot-natured Media

Chinese onion juice   Cut the onion (with the root) into
small pieces, squeeze, then dilute with water in equal
proportions.
Nature and taste   Warm and pungent.
Functions   Induce sweating and relieve Exterior Syndrome; promote Yang and reduce edema.
Applications   Common cold marked by headache,
chills, fever and stuffed nose when used at Fengchi (GB
20), Dazhui (DU 14) and Yingxiang (LI 20). Pain in
the lower abdomen and oliguria when used at Shenque
(REN 8) and on the lower abdomen.
Ginger juice   Finely grate fresh ginger, squeeze, then

15

dilute with water in equal proportions.

Nature and taste   Slightly warm and pungent.

Functions   Expel Wind and disperse Cold; warm the Middle Jiao and relieve vomiting.

Applications   Prevent and treat common cold, cold sensation in the upper back, stiffness of the neck, headache without sweating, cough with sputum and asthma when used at some points in the neck, upper back and along the spine; strengthen the therapeutic effect of manipulations for abdominal pain and diarrhea when used on the abdomen.

Huoxiang (Herba Agastachis) juice   Crush fresh agastache leaves and stems into pulp, then dilute with water in equal proportion.

Nature and taste   Slightly warm and pungent.

Functions   Relieve Summer Heat and remove Damp; regulate Qi and mediate the Middle Jiao.

Applications   Prevent and treat headache and dizziness due to Summer Heat when used on the indicated points in the head; relieve oppression and fullness in the chest, nausea and vomiting when used on the abdomen.

Sesame oil

Nature and taste   Slightly warm, sweet and bland.

Functions   Reduce weakness and strengthen the Spleen; moisten Dryness.

Applications   Prevent and treat malnutrition, Spleen and Stomach Deficiency Syndromes and dry skin when used at relevant points.

Cold and Cool-natured Media

Peppermint juice   Crush fresh mint leaves and stems into pulp, then dilute with water in equal proportions.

Nature and taste   Cold and pungent.

16

Functions   Expel Wind and reduce fever; relieve depression and treat Exterior Syndrome.

Applications   Relieve common cold due to Wind Heat, and rubella when used at certain points on the head and hands.

Cold water

Nature and taste   Cool and sweet.

Functions   Clear Heat and relieve fever.

Applications   Enhance the function of relieving high fever when used at points on the hands.

Talcum powder   Known as Huashi when used dissolved in water.

Nature and taste   Cold, bland and sweet.

Functions   Clear Heat and remove Damp; smooth the skin and protect it during manipulations.

Applications   Talcum powder can be used on all parts of the body for all disorders.

Milk

Nature and taste   Bland, sweet and salty.

Functions   Reduce weakness and tonify Qi; clear Heat and moisten Dryness; benefit five Zang Organs; nourish Yin and Blood; promote Heart Qi; regulate digestion.

Applications   Prevent and treat abdominal distention and pain, malnutrition, diarrhea and retention of urine when used on the abdomen; tonify weakness and clear Heat when used on any part of the body.

Basic
Manipulations

Pushing (Tui Fa)

Pressing directly with the pad of the thumb, or those of the index and middle fingers together.

Key points Keep the shoulders relaxed and low, the elbow bent, the wrist straight. Induce force into the forearm, then push in the specified direction.

Pushing with the thumb Induce force into the pad or lateral side of the thumb (see Fig. 2-1,2).

Site: Head, face, chest, abdomen, lumbar area, back and limbs.

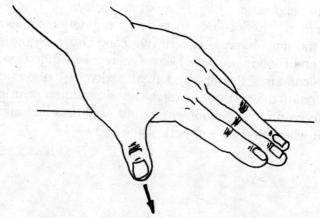

Fig. 2-1   Pushing with the thumb (Vertical pushing)

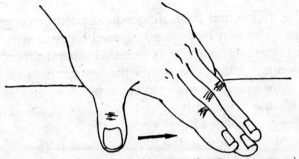
Fig. 2-2   Pushing with the thumb (Horizontal pushing)

Pushing with two fingers   Induce force into the pads of the index and middle fingers (see Fig. 2-3).
Site: Forearm, spine and back.

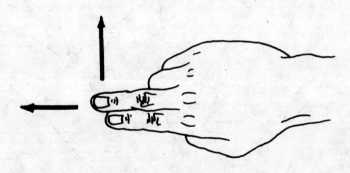
Fig. 2-3   Pushing with two fingers

Therapeutic actions   Activate channels and collaterals, stop pain and relieve spasm; promote the circulation

19

of Qi and Blood, balance Yin and Yang.

Grasping (Na Fa)

Use the thumb and index finger in opposition to grasp and lift (The ring finger may be used together with the index finger). The action is repeated several times.

Key points   Induce force into the tips or pads of fingers. Care should be taken to avoid pinching and marking with the fingernails. Wrist joint should coordinate with the movement of the finger joints. Grasp the muscle, joint or point with the thumb against fingers.

Grasping with two fingers   The thumb and index fingers are in opposition. Induce force into the tips of these fingers (see Fig. 2-4).

Site: The back of neck, the ends of limbs.

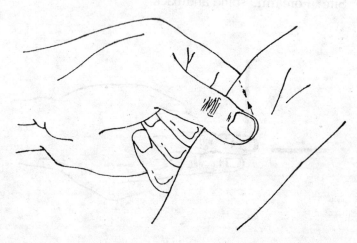

Fig. 2-4   Grasping with two fingers

Grasping with four fingers   The thumb in opposition to the index, middle and ring fingers. Induce force into

20

the tips of the fingers (see Fig. 2-5).
Site: Lumbar area, abdomen, large muscles on limbs (e.g., biceps, quadriceps).

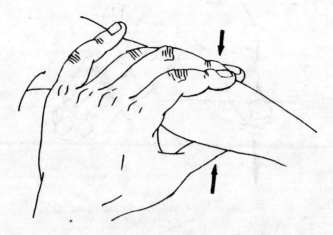

Fig. 2-5   Grasping with four fingers

Therapeutic actions   Induce sweating and relieve Exterior Syndrome; open orifices and clear the Mind; regulate the circulation of Qi and Blood; relax tendons and activate collaterals; relieve spasm and check convulsion.

Pressing (An Fa)

Place the thumb or palm on the specified area or point, then press with increasing force.
Key points   Press deeply with even and gentle pressure. The action is rhythmically repeated.
Pressing with the finger   With the thumb or middle finger straight and other fingers bent, induce force into the thumb or middle finger (see Fig. 2-6,7).

21

Site: All parts or points of the body.

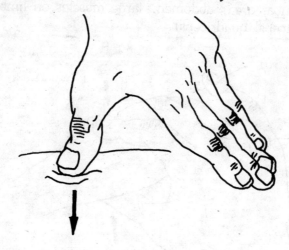

Fig. 2-6   Pressing with the thumb

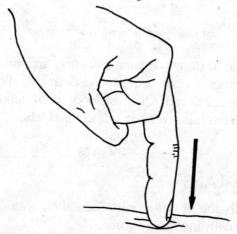

Fig. 2-7   Pressing with the middle finger

Pressing with the palm   With the arm straight and wrist extended, induce force into the base of the palm, or the thenar or hypothenar eminence (see Fig. 2-8).

22

Site: Lumbar area, back and abdomen.

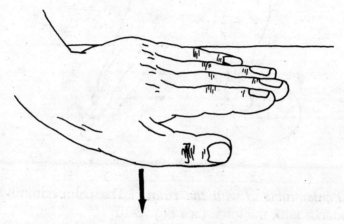

Fig. 2-8 Pressing with the palm

Therapeutic actions Warm channels and activate the collaterals, relieve fright and relax spasm; promote the circulation of Qi and Blood and regulate the tendons.

Circular Rubbing (Mo Fa)

Use the finger or palm to rub gently and rhythmically over the area with a circular motion.

Key points Keeping the shoulders relaxed and low, and the wrist free and loose, induce force into the forearm. The manipulation should be smoothly and evenly performed on the skin surface, without moving the underlying muscles.

Circular rubbing with the finger Using the the thumb or index, middle and ring fingers together, induce force into the pads (see Fig. 2-9).

Site: Head, face, chest and abdomen.

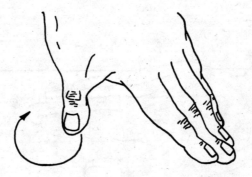

Fig. 2-9   Circular rubbing with the thumb

Circular rubbing with the palm   The palm naturally extends with the force (see Fig. 2-10).
Site: Lumbar area, back and abdomen.

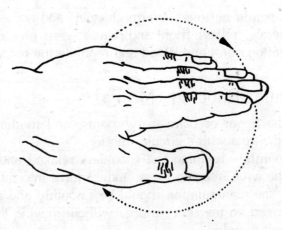

Fig. 2-10   Circular rubbing with the palm

Therapeutic actions   Mediate the Middle Jiao and regulate the flow of Qi; strengthen the Spleen and regulate the Stomach; promote the circulation of Qi and Blood to remove Blood Stasis, relieve pain and relax spasm.

Kneading (Rou Fa)

Gently and flexibly move the pads of the fingers or the whole palm in a circle.

Key points The shoulders should be relaxed and low with the arm bent. Induce force into the forearm and wrist. The movement is circular, deep and gentle, so the underlying tissue moves. Gliding and rubbing over the skin should be avoided.

Kneading with single finger Knead with the thumb with other fingers in a loose fist (see Fig. 2-11). Or knead with middle finger with other fingers in a loose fist (see Fig. 2-12).

Site: Head, face, neck, chest, abdomen and limbs.

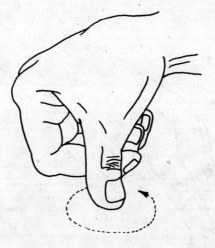

Fig. 2-11 Kneading with the thumb

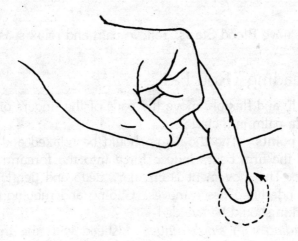

Fig. 2-12   Kneading with the middle finger

Kneading with two fingers   Induce force into the index and middle fingers with other fingers bent, then knead in a circle (see Fig. 2-13).
Site: Shoulders, along spine, lumbar area and buttocks.

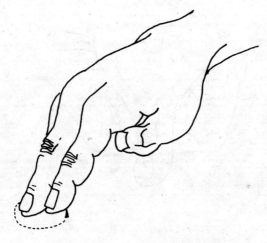

Fig. 2-13   Kneading with two fingers

26

Kneading with the thenar eminence (*base of the thumb*) Induce force into the thenar area, then knead in a circle (see Fig 2-14).
Site: Head, face, chest and abdomen.

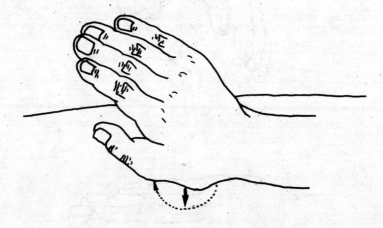

Fig. 2-14   Kneading with the thenar eminence

Kneading with the hypothenar eminence (*side of palm below little finger*) Induce force into the hypothenar eminence, then knead in a circle (see Fig. 2-15).
Site: The back of the neck, shoulders, back and lumbosacral area.
Kneading with the palm Induce force into the hand, then knead in a circle (see Fig. 2-16).
Site: Lumbar area, back, abdomen and limbs.

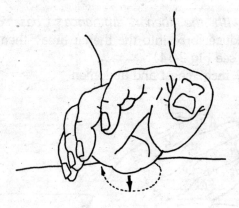

Fig. 2-15   Kneading with the hypothenar eminence

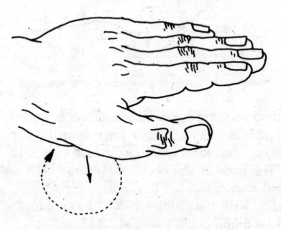

Fig. 2-16   Kneading with the palm

Therapeutic actions   Promote the circulation of Qi and Blood and remove Stagnation; disperse accumulation and activate collaterals; relax tendons and ease the joints.

Circular Gliding (Yun Fa)

Glide in a circular motion with either thumb or middle finger. The movement is repeated with pressure.

Key points   With the shoulders and the wrist relaxed, the elbow flexed, and the thumb extended, induce force into the tip or radial border of the manipulating finger with other fingers in a loose fist, then knead in a broad circular motion with pressure (see Fig. 2-17, 18).

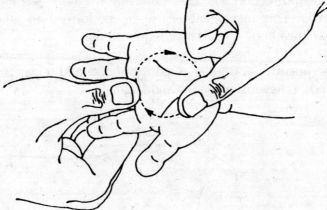

Fig. 2-17   Circular gliding Bagua (Yun Bagua)

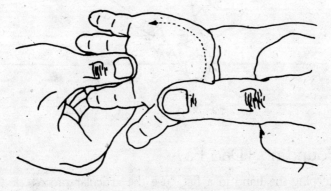

Fig. 2-18   Circular gliding Earth (Spleen)
into Water (Kidney) (Yunturushui)

Site Hand and some points in the head.
Therapeutic actions Regulate Qi and Blood; activate the channels and collaterals.

Marking (Qia Fa)

Use one thumbnail to press the skin.
Key points Concentrate force into the thumbnail in a vertical direction but do not damage the skin (see Fig. 2-19). This movement is usually performed together with kneading, i. e. "kneading-marking."
Site Any point of the body.
Therapeutic actions Open orifices and clear the Mind; relieve convulsions and fright.

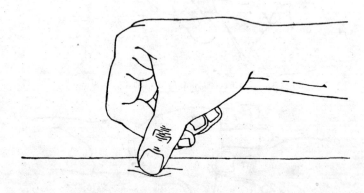

Fig. 2-19 Marking with the thumbnail

Pounding (Dao Fa)

Keeping the hand in a fist, use the articular process or the tip of one finger to pound the specified point rhythmically.
Key points This motion is done from the elbow rather

than the wrist, and should be done at a frequency of 150 times per minute.

Pounding with the articular process (finger joint)   The hand is in a fist with the middle finger flexed as shown in Fig. 2-20. Induce force into the flexed joint to pound the specified point.

Site: Points in the hand.

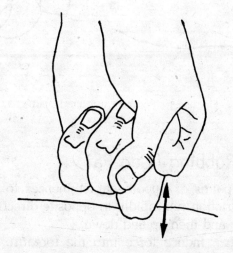

Fig. 2-20   Pounding with the articular process

Pounding with the fingertip   With the middle finger supported by thumb and index fingers together, induce force into the middle finger to pound with the fingertip (see Fig. 2-21).

Site: Points in head and face.

Therapeutic actions   Open the orifices and clear the Mind; relieve fright and calm the Mind; relieve spasm and stop pain.

31

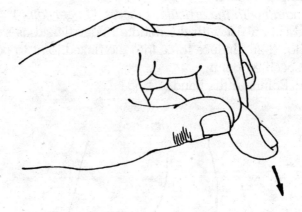

Fig. 2-21   Pounding with the fingertip

Piston Rubbing (Cuo Fa)

Use both palms or hypothenar eminences to hold the area and friction rub rapidly in opposite directions back and forth, and then up and down.

Key points   Induce force into the forearm. Keeping both wrists and fingers naturally extended, rub evenly and flexibly to generate heat (see Fig. 2-22).

Site   Lumbar area (piston rubbing with the whole palm), and limbs (piston rubbing with the thenar eminences).

Therapeutic actions   Warm the channels and activate the collaterals; expel Wind and disperse Cold; soothe the Liver and regulate Qi; promote digestion.

32

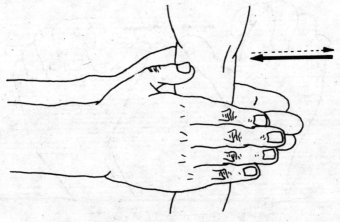

Fig. 2-22   Piston rubbing

Convergently and Divergently Pushing (He, Fen Fa)

Beginning at two separate points along skin and pushing both thumbs toward a common point in the middle is called convergent pushing (see Fig. 2-23). Beginning at a common point and pushing both thumbs evenly to separated points is called divergent pushing (see Fig. 2-24).

Key points   Keeping the elbow flexed and the wrist extended, extend both thumbs with other fingers clenched; induce force into the wrist and fingers to push.

Site   Points in wrist, chest and abdomen.

Therapeutic actions   Promote the circulation of Qi and Blood, balance Yin and Yang, relax the chest and regulate Qi (convergent pushing); regulate the circulation of Qi and Blood, mediate Yin and Yang (divergent pushing).

33

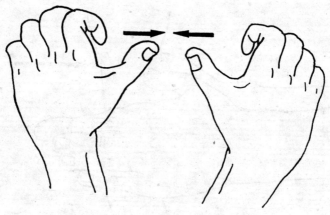

Fig. 2-23   Convergently pushing

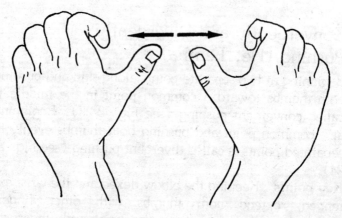

Fig. 2-24   Divergently pushing

Pinching and Lifting Along both Sides of the Spine (Nie Ji Fa)

Pinch and lift the skin along both sides of the spine. The hands should move alternately, beginning at the base of the spine and working their way up.

34

Key points   Both thumbs extended, and other fingers loosely clenched. Either the thumbs and the index fingers only may be used (see Fig. 2-25) or use the thumbs and the index and middle fingers (see Fig. 2-26). Start in the lower lumbar area and pinch upward toward the neck. After every third pinch, twist and tug the skin upward.

Site   Back from Guiwei to Dazhui (DU 14).

Therapeutic actions   Regulate Yin and Yang, calm the Mind and benefit the brain; promote the circulation of Qi, Blood and Zangfu; regulate the Stomach and strengthen the Spleen and promote digestion.

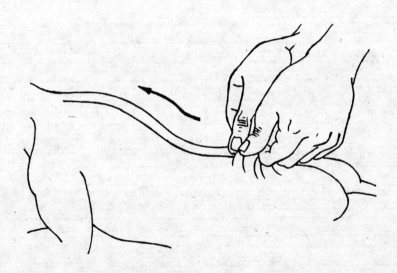

Fig. 2-25   Pinching and lifting along
both sides of the spine (1)

35

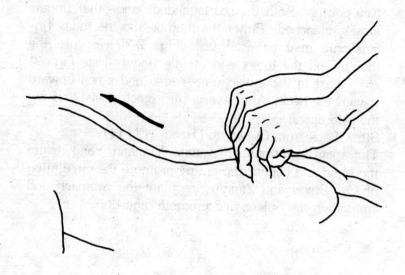

Fig. 2-26   Pinching and lifting along
both sides of the spine (2)

36

COMMONLY
USED SEQUENCES

The Head and Neck

Circular Gliding Taiyang (Yun Taiyang)

Site In the depression posterior to the midpoint between the outer canthus and the lateral end of the eyebrow.

Procedure The child sits or lies face up. Hold his head with index, middle and ring fingers of both hands. Circular glide Taiyang (Extra) with both thumbs (see Fig. 3-1). Work forward to reinforce, and the reverse to reduce. Repeat the movement 20 to 50 times.

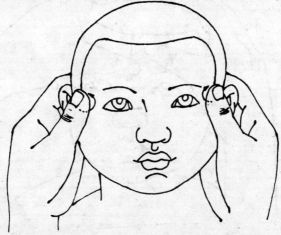

Fig. 3-1 Circular gliding Taiyang

Therapeutic actions   Expel Wind and clear Heat, open the orifices and relieve fright.

Indications   Convulsion, fever, irritability, Exterior Syndrome without sweating, headache and pain in the eyes.

Opening Tianmen (Kai Tianmen)

Site   The line between the eyebrows and extending up along the middle of the forehead to the anterior hairline.

Procedure   The child sits or lies face up. Each hand supports his head with index, middle and ring fingers together. Alternating thumbs, push in a straight line with the pad or radial edge, from Yintang (Extra) up to the anterior hairline (see Fig. 3-2). Repeat 30 to 50 times.

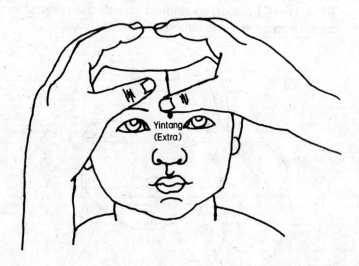

Fig. 3-2 Opening Tianmen

Therapeutic actions   Expel Wind and relieve Exterior Syndrome, open the orifices and clear the Mind, calm the Mind and relieve fright.

Indications   Convulsion, palpitation due to fright, common cold marked by fever, headache and dizziness.

Pushing Kangong (Tui Kangong)

Site   The line starting from one cun above the center point between the eyebrows and extending along the forehead above and parallel to the eyebrows.

Procedure   Hold the infant's head with both hands and mark divergently with the thumbnails along Kangong, then push divergently with the radial edge of the thumbs from Yintang (Extra) along the eyebrows to Taiyang (Extra) 30 to 50 times (see Fig. 3-3).

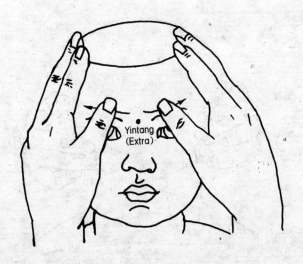

Fig. 3-3   Pushing Kangong

Therapeutic actions Expel Wind and disperse Cold, open the orifices and clear the Mind.

Indications Convulsion, headache, painful bloodshot eyes and high fever with upward staring.

Circular Gliding Erhougaogu (Yun Erhougaogu)

Site On the mastoid process behind Yifeng (SJ 17).

Procedure Support the infant's head with the thumb, index and ring fingers of both hands and glide over the point in a circular motion using the middle finger. Glide forward to reinforce and the reverse to reduce. Repeat 20 to 50 times (see Fig. 3-4).

Therapeutic actions Clear Heat and disperse Wind, calm the Mind and relieve fright.

Indications Headache, convulsion and irritability.

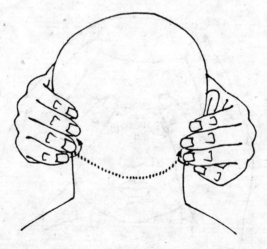

Fig. 3-4   Circular gliding Erhougaogu

Pushing Fontanel (Tui Xinmen)

Site In the depression below Baihui (DU 20) on the midline.

Procedure Supporting the infant's head with the index, middle and ring fingers of both hands, push alternately from the anterior hairline to Xinmen with both thumbs 30 to 50 times, then push divergently from Xinmen to both sides of the head 20 to 30 times. If the fontanel has not closed, this manipulation should be done carefully and gently only to the lower border. Pressing should be avoided (see Fig. 3-5).

Therapeutic actions Disperse Wind and relieve fright, open the orifices and clear the Mind, strengthen the brain and improve mentality.

Indications Convulsion marked by staring upward; Exterior Syndrome marked by stuffed and running nose.

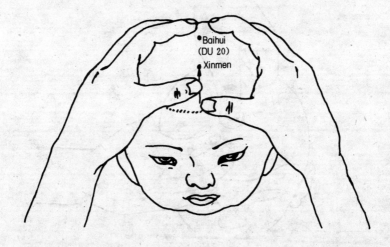

Fig. 3-5 Pushing Xinmen

Kneading Baihui (Rou Baihui DU 2)

Site The center of the top of the head: the intersection of the midline with a line drawn from the apex of each ear.

Procedure The child's head is supported with the left hand while the point is marked 3 to 5 times and then kneaded 30 to 50 times using the right hand (see Fig. 3-6).

Therapeutic actions Lift Yang and reduce Qi Sinking, calm the Mind and relieve fright; open the orifices and improve vision, strengthen the brain and benefit mentality.

Indications Convulsion, headache, dizziness, prolapse of the anus, diarrhea and bed-wetting.

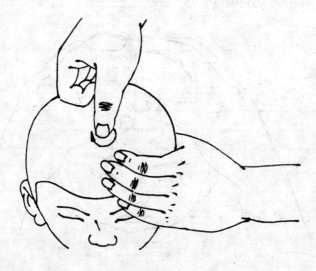

Fig. 3-6   Kneading Baihui

44

Kneading Sishencong (Rou Sishencong)

Site 1 cun below and above, lateral to Baihui (DU 20).

Procedure Holding the infant's head with the fingers of both hands, knead the four points with the thumbs 30 to 50 times for each point (see Fig. 3-7).

Therapeutic actions Strengthen the brain and benefit mentality, calm the Mind and relieve fright, alleviate pain.

Indications Headache, dizziness, dim eyesight, restlessness and epilepsy.

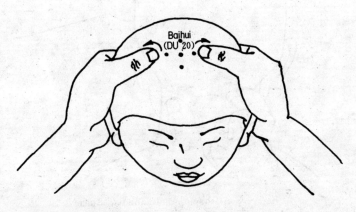

Fig. 3-7 Kneading Sishencong

Grasping and Kneading Fengchi (Na Rou Fengchi GB 2)

Site In the depression immediately below the occipital bone.

Procedure Supporting the infant's head with one

45

hand, place the thumb and index finger of the other hand against the points on the opposite sides of the neck, grasp three times, then knead 10 to 30 times (see Fig. 3-8). This manipulation should be gently performed because the points are sensitive.

Therapeutic actions   Expel Wind and improve vision, induce sweating and alleviate pain.

Indications   Headache, dizziness and fever without sweating.

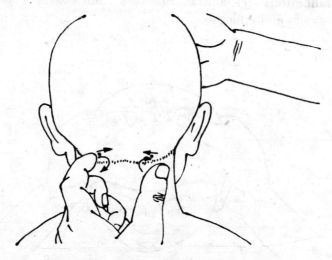

Fig. 3-8   Grasping and kneading Baihui

Kneading Dazhui (Rou Dazhui DU 14)

Site   Between the seventh cervical vertebra and the first thoracic vertebra.

Procedure   The child sits or lies face down. Knead the point while pressing with the thumb or the middle finger 30 to 50 times (see Fig. 3-9).

46

Therapeutic actions   Raise Yang Qi and treat Exterior Syndrome by inducing sweating; improve asthma and relieve vomiting, clear Heat and check Wind, relax spasm and alleviate pain.

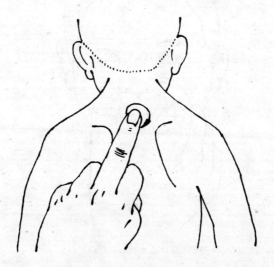

Fig. 3-9   Kneading Dazhui

Indications   Exterior Syndrome marked by fever, stiff neck, asthma, vomiting, diarrhea and convulsion.

Kneading Yingxiang
(Rou Yingxiang LI 2)

Site   In the nasolabial groove, level with the midpoint of the lateral border of the alae nasi.

Procedure   Supporting the infant's head with one hand, knead the points with the thumb and index finger, or the index and middle fingers of the other hand 50 to 80 times (see Fig. 3-10).

Therapeutic actions   Open the orifices and clear the

47

Mind.
Indications   Deviation of the eyes and mouth, nose-bleed, stuffed and running nose.

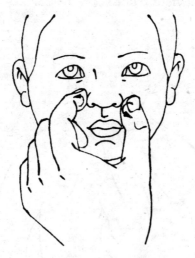

Fig. 3-10   Kneading Yingxiang

Ape Picking up Fruit
(Yuan Hou Zhai Guo)

Site   The apex and lobe of both ears.
Procedure   Pinch both ear apexes longitudinally with the index and middle fingers and lift 10 to 20 times, then pinch both earlobes and pull downward 10 to 20 times (see Fig. 3-11).
Therapeutic actions   Relieve convulsion and calm the Mind, regulate Qi and remove Phlegm, strengthen the Spleen and promote digestion.
Indications   Convulsion, headache, dizziness, cough, asthma, diarrhea and prolapse of the anus.

48

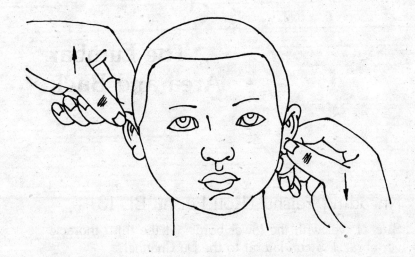

Fig. 3-11 Ape picking up fruit

The Lumbar Area and Back

Kneading Feishu (Rou Feishu BL 13)

Site   Level with the lower border of the third thoracic vertebra, 1.5 cun lateral to the Du Channel.

Procedure   Knead the points with both thumbs or the index and middle fingers together 50 to 100 times. Knead medially to reinforce, and the reverse to reduce. Reinforcing is used for Deficiency Syndrome, and reducing is used for Excess Syndrome (see Fig. 3-12).

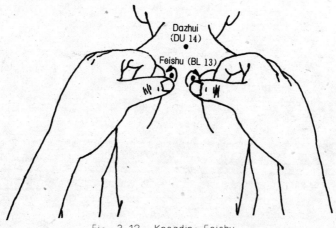

Fig. 3-12   Kneading Feishu

Therapeutic actions Tonify Lung Qi, regulate the flow of Qi and alleviate pain; relieve cough by descending Lung Qi.

Indications Cough, asthma, fullness and oppression of the chest due to Lung Heat; cough due to invasion of Wind Cold and cough due to Deficiency of Lung Qi.

Kneading Ganshu (Rou Ganshu BL 18)

Site Level with the lower border of the ninth thoracic vertebra, 1.5 cun lateral to the Du Channel.

Procedure Knead the points with both thumbs or the index and middle fingers together 50 to 100 times. Knead medially to reinforce, and the reverse to reduce. Reducing is more frequently used than reinforcing (see Fig. 3-13).

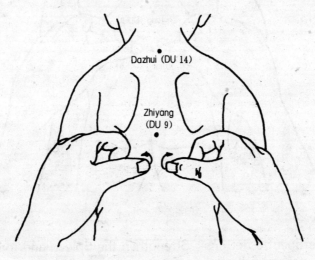

Dazhui (DU 14)

Zhiyang
(DU 9)

Fig. 3-13 Kneading Ganshu

Therapeutic actions   Soothe the Liver and regulate Liver Qi; clear the Liver and improve vision.

Indications   Pain in the hypochondria due to stagnation of Liver Qi; painful bloodshot eyes; headache and dizziness.

Kneading Pishu (Rou Pishu BL 2)

Site   Level with the lower border of the eleventh thoracic vertebra, 1.5 cun lateral to the Du Channel.

Procedure   Knead with both thumbs or the index and middle fingers together 50 to 100 times. Knead medially to reinforce, and the reverse to reduce. Reinforcing is more frequently used than reducing (see Fig. 3-14).

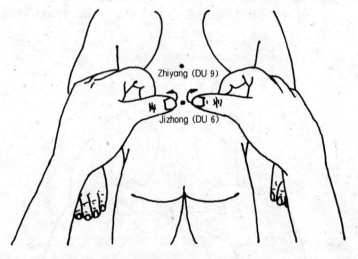

Fig. 3-14 Kneading Pishu

Therapeutic actions   Strengthen the Spleen and tonify Qi; promote digestion.

Indications   Malnutrition due to Deficiency of Middle

52

Qi, loss of appetite, vomiting, diarrhea and prolapse.

Kneading Weishu (Rou Weishu BL 21)

Site Level with the lower border of twelfth thoracic vertebra, 1.5 cun lateral to the Du Channel.

Procedure Knead with both thumbs or the index and middle fingers together 50 to 100 times. Knead medially to reinforce, and the reverse to reduce. Reducing is more frequently used than reinforcing (see Fig. 3-15).

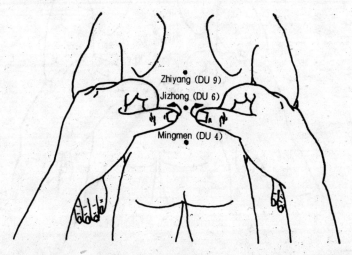

Fig. 3-15 Kneading Weishu

Therapeutic actions Strengthen the Stomach, promote digestion and improve appetite.

Indications Pain and distention in the upper abdomen, malnutrition, loss of appetite, vomiting and diarrhea.

53

Kneading Shenshu (Rou Shenshu BL 23)

Site Level with the lower border of the second lumbar vertebra, 1.5 cun lateral to the Du Channel.

Procedure Knead with both thumbs or the index and middle fingers together 50 to 100 times. Knead medially to reinforce, and the reverse to reduce. Reinforcing is more commonly used (see Fig. 3-16).

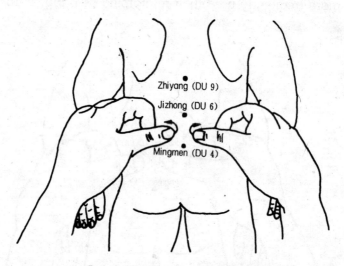

Fig. 3-16 Kneading Shenshu

Therapeutic actions Reinforce the Kidney and benefit mentality; strengthen lumbar area and knees, relax ligaments, tendons and muscles by tonifying primordial Qi.

Indications Five kinds of flaccidity and retardation and weak mentality, pain in lumbar area and bed-wetting.

54

Kneading Guiwei (Rou Guiwei)

Site   Midway between the coccyx and the anus.
Procedure   The child lies face down. Knead Guiwei with the thumb or the index and middle fingers together 100 to 500 times (see Fig. 3-17).
Therapeutic actions   Promote the Qi of the Du Channel; regulate the functions of the Large Intestine; relieve fright and calm the Mind; induce constipation and stop diarrhea.
Indications   Constipation, diarrhea, prolapse of the anus and infantile convulsion.

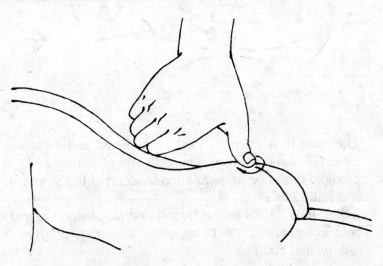

Fig. 3-17   Kneading Guiwei

Pushing the Upper Back (Tui Bei Lei)

Site   The area from Dazhui (DU 14) to the level of the second lumbar vertebra.
Procedure   The child lies face down. Extend both

hands naturally, place both palms on the back to push down 50 to 100 times (see Fig. 3-18).

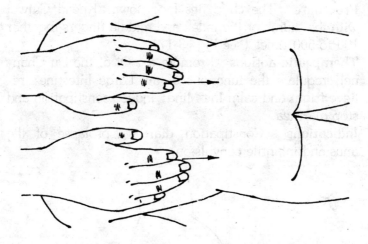

Fig. 3-18   Pushing the upper back

Therapeutic actions   Soothe the Liver and regulate Liver Qi; remove Phlegm by activating the flow of Qi; promote digestion by regulating function of the Stomach and Intestines.

Indications   Pain in the hypochondria, distention and pain in abdomen, loss of appetite, vomiting, diarrhea, asthma and cough.

Pinching and Lifting Along both Sides of the Spine (Nie Ji)

See Page 34 and Fig. 3-19.

56

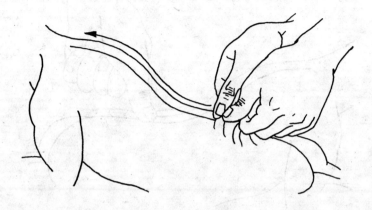

Fig. 3-19 · Pinching and lifting along
both sides of the spine

The Pushing Qijiegu (Tui Qijiegu)

Site   The line along the spine and head from Mingmen
(DU 4) to Chengjiang (REN 24).

Procedure   Push with the thumb. Reinforce by pushing
upward, reduce by pushing downward (see Fig. 3-20).
Repeat the motion 100 times.

Therapeutic actions   Warm Yang and relieve diarrhea
if pushing upward; purge Heat, relax the bowel and descend rebellious Qi if pushing downward.

Indications   Diarrhea or chronic dysentery with prolapse of the anus if pushing upward; constipation, dry
stools if pushing downward.

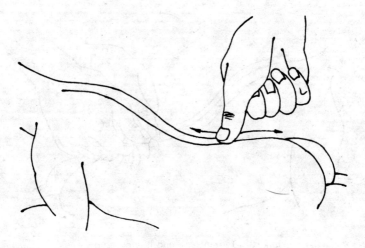

Fig. 3-20   Pushing Qijiegu

58

The Posterior Lower Limbs

Pressing and Kneading Huantiao (An Rou Huantiao GB 3)

Site At the junction of the lateral 1/3 and medial 2/3 of the distance between the greater trochanter and the hiatus of the sacrum (Yaoshu DU 2). The child should be semi-prone with thigh straight.

Procedure Press the point with the thumb 3 to 5 times, then knead while pressing 50 to 100 times (see Fig. 3-21).

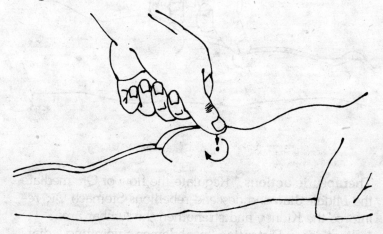

Fig. 3-21 Pressing and kneading Huantiao

Therapeutic actions Purge Liver and Gallbladder Fire; activate the channels and alleviate pain.
Indications Headache, bloodshot eyes and flaccidity of the lower limbs.

Pressing and Kneading Weizhong (An Rou Weizhong BL 4)

Site In the center of the popliteal fossa.
Procedure Press the point 3 to 5 times, then knead 50 to 100 times (see Fig. 3-22).

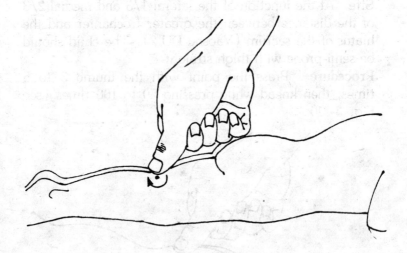

Fig 3-22 Pressing and kneading Weizhong

Therapeutic actions Regulate the flow of Qi, mediate the Middle Jiao and descend rebellious Stomach Qi; reinforce the Kidney and strengthen the lumbar area.
Indications Distention in abdomen, vomiting, diarrhea and bed-wetting.

Grasping Chengshan
(Na Chengshan BL 57)

Site Directly inferior to the belly of the gastrocnemius muscle, at the point where the muscle divides.

Procedure Place the thumb on the point with the other fingers placed on the anterior shin in opposition to the thumb. Knead while grasping 3 to 5 times (see Fig. 3-23).

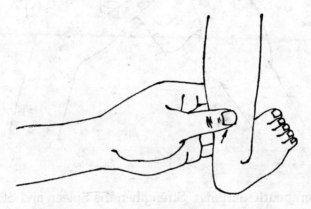

Fig. 3-23   Grasping Chengshan

Therapeutic actions Activate the channels and collaterals; relax the tendons and promote circulation; relieve fright and calm the Mind.

Indications Convulsion, constipation, prolapse of the anus, vomiting, diarrhea and flaccidity of the lower limbs.

Kneading Sanyinjiao
(Rou Sanyinjiao)

Site 3 cun directly above the tip of the medial malleo-

61

lus, on the posterior border of the tibia.

Procedure Knead the point 30 to 50 times (see Fig. 3-24).

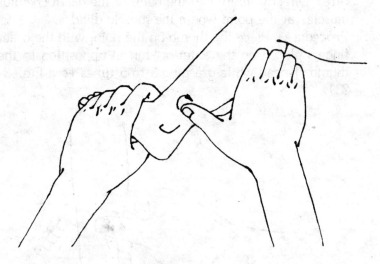

Fig. 3-24 Kneading Sanyinjiao

Therapeutic actions Strengthen the Spleen and Stomach; nourish the Heart and Kidney, promote metabolism of Body Fluids.

Indications Convulsion, spasm, pain and distention in abdomen, diarrhea, constipation, insomnia with palpitation due to fright and bed-wetting.

Kneading and Friction Rubbing Yongquan (Rou Ca Yongquan KID 1)

Site On the midline of the sole of the foot at the junction of the anterior 1/3 and posterior 2/3.

Procedure Knead with the thumb or the middle finger 30 to 50 times, then rub with the thumb from the big

62

toe to the heel. The motion is rapidly repeated until heat is produced (see Fig. 3-25).

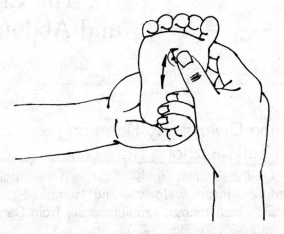

Fig. 3-25   Kneading and friction rubbing Yongquan

Therapeutic actions   Clear the Mind and descend rebellious Qi; nourish the Kidney and benefit the brain; clear Heat and relieve irritability.

Indications   Headache, dizziness, fever with restlessness, convulsion, five palm heat and insomnia with irritability.

The Chest
and Abdomen

Pushing Divergently Danzhong
(Fen Tui Danzhong REN 17)

Site   On the sternum, midway between the nipples.
Procedure   Push divergently and laterally 50 to 100 times with both thumbs simultaneously from Danzhong to the nipples (see Fig. 3-26).

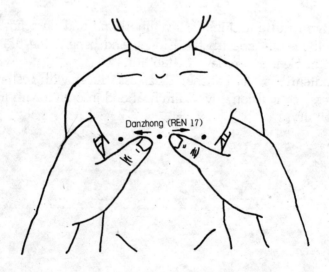

Fig. 3-26   Pushing divergently Danzhong

Therapeutic actions   Soothe the chest and regulate the flow of Qi; benefit the Heart and relieve irritability; improve asthma and stop cough.

Indications   Oppression of the chest, shortness of breath, palpitation, cough, asthma and vomiting.

Kneading Rupang (Rou Rupang)

Site   0.2 cun lateral to the nipples.

Procedure   Knead with the thumb or the index finger 50 to 100 times (see Fig. 3-27).

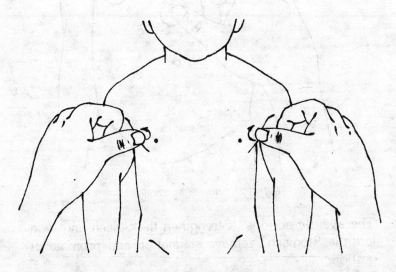

Fig. 3-27   Kneading Rupang

Therapeutic actions   Soothe the chest and regulate the flow of Qi; remove Phlegm and stop cough.

Indications   Oppression of the chest, cough with rales and vomiting.

Kneading Zhongwan
(Rou Zhongwan REN 12)

Site Midway between the umbilicus and xiphoid process.

Procedure Knead the point with the thumb or the index finger 200 to 500 times (see Fig. 3-28).

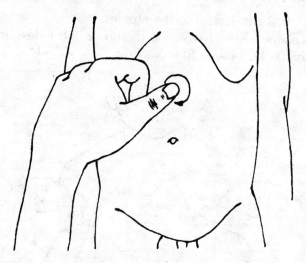

Fig. 3-28 Kneading Zhongwan

Therapeutic actions Strengthen the Spleen and regulate the Stomach, remove stagnation and promote digestion.

Indications Pain and distention of the abdomen, vomiting and loss of appetite.

Circular Gliding Shenque
(Mo Sheque REN 8)

Site In the center of the umbilicus.

66

Procedure   Glide with the whole palm or the index, middle and ring fingers together 100 to 300 times in a circular motion (see Fig. 3-29).

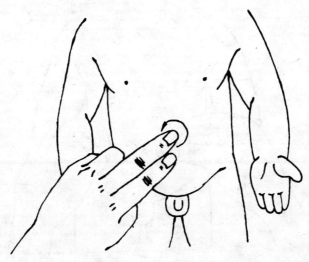

Fig. 3-29 · Circular gliding Shenque

Therapeutic actions   Mediate the Middle Jiao and regulate Stomach Qi, remove stagnation and promote digestion.

Indications   Distention of the abdomen, borborygmus, diarrhea due to food stagnation, constipation and malnutrition.

Kneading Tianshu (Rou Tianshu ST 25)

Site   2 cun lateral to the umbilicus.

Procedure   Knead with the index and middle fingers together 30 to 50 times (see Fig 3-30).

Therapeutic actions   Regulate the flow of Qi and alleviate pain; induce diuresis and relieve edema; promote

67

digestion and benefit the Large Intestine.
Indications Diarrhea with bowel sounds, distention of the abdomen, constipation and edema.

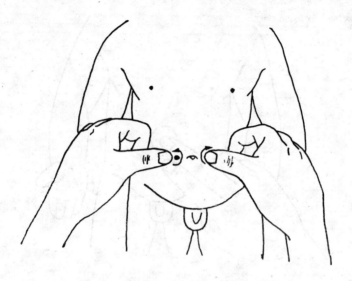

Fig. 3-30   Kneading Tianshu

Circular Gliding Dantian (Mo Dantian Extra)

Site 2-3 cun below the umbilicus in the middle of the lower abdomen.

Procedure Circular gliding with the palm or the index, middle and ring fingers together 100 to 500 times (see Fig 3-31).

Therapeutic actions Warm and reinforce Kidney Yang; alleviate pain and induce diuresis.

Indications Pain in the lower abdomen, constipation, diarrhea, bed-wetting and prolapse of the anus.

68

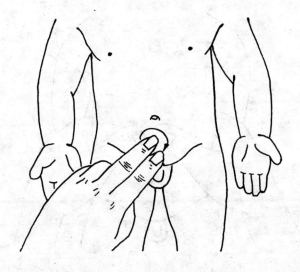

Fig. 3-31 Circular gliding Dantian

Separating Yin and Yang of the Abdomen (Fen Fu Yin Yang)

Site The area from the hypochondria to the hips.

Procedure Push divergently with both thumbs along each side of the inferior border of the floating twelfth rib 100 to 300 times (see Fig. 3-32).

Therapeutic actions Remove stagnation and relieve distention; regulate the flow of Qi and alleviate pain; descend rebellious Qi and relieve vomiting.

Indications Food stagnation, distention of the abdomen, vomiting, loss of appetite and malnutrition.

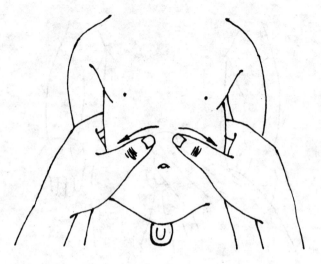

Fig. 3-32   Separating Yin and Yang of the abdomen

Pressing and Rubbing down the Sides of the Body (An Xuan Zou Cuo Mo)

Site   The area from under the armpits to the hips.

Procedure   Put both hands under the child's armpits with thumbs pointing up to press the chest, then slide both hands down the infant's sides to the hips (see Fig. 3-33). Repeat the motion 5 to 10 times.

Therapeutic actions   Regulate the flow of Qi and remove Phlegm; descend rebellious Qi and relieve vomiting.

Indications   Oppression of the chest, asthma, cough, vomiting, pain and distention of the hypochondria and abdomen due to accumulation of Phlegm or stagnation of Qi.

70

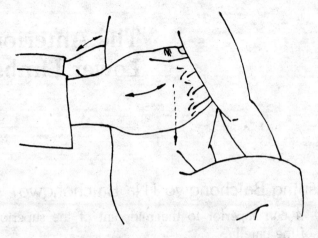

Fig. 3-33 Pressing and rubbing down
the sides of the body

The Anterior
Lower Limbs

Grasping Baichongwo (Na Baichongwo)

Site   4 cun superior to the midpoint of the superior edge of the patella.

Procedure   Grasp while pinching the points on both legs between the index and middle fingers 3 to 5 times (see Fig. 3-34).

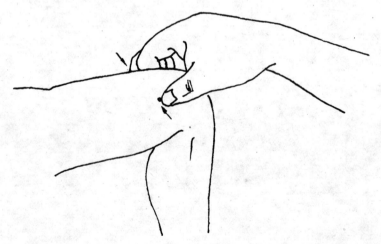

Fig. 3-34   Grasping Baichongwo

Therapeutic actions   Tranquilize the Mind and relieve

fright; expel Wind and activate the collaterals.

Indications Convulsion, spasm, coma, rubella and itching of the skin.

Kneading While Pressing Zusanli (An Rou Zusanli ST 36)

Site 3 cun inferior to the lateral Guiyan point, 1 cun lateral to the tibia.

Procedure Knead while pressing the point with the thumb or middle finger (see Fig. 3-35). Repeat the motion 100 to 300 times for treating a disorder; 500 to 800 times for enhancing body resistance.

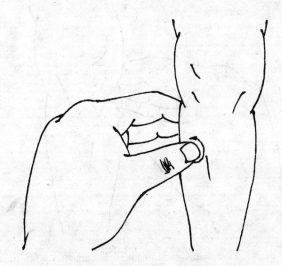

Fig. 3-35 Kneading while pressing Zusanli

Therapeutic actions Regulate the flow of Qi and mediate the Middle Jiao; benefit the brain and clear the Mind; strengthen the Spleen and regulate the Stomach; promote digestion and descend rebellious Qi.

73

Indications Distention and pain of the abdomen, nausea, vomiting, hiccups, loss of appetite, malnutrition, diarrhea, dysentery or constipation; headache, dizziness, insomnia, asthma and listlessness.

Kneading Yanglingquan
(Rou Yanglingquan GB 34)

Site In the depression anterior and inferior to the head of the fibula.
Procedure Knead the point with the thumb or tip of the middle finger 50 to 100 times (see Fig. 3-36).

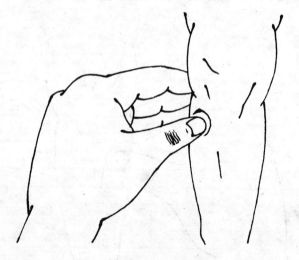

Fig. 3-36 Kneading Yanglingquan

Therapeutic actions Soothe the Liver and regulate Liver Qi; promote the channels and collaterals.
Indications Headache, dizziness, pain in the hypochondria, vomiting, constipation; flaccidity of the lower limbs.

Kneading Guiyan (Rou Guiyan)

Site The two depressions on the inferior edge of the patella, medial and lateral to the patellar ligament, located with the knee flexed.

Procedure Knead the point with the thumb or the index and middle fingers together 30 to 50 times (see Fig. 3-37).

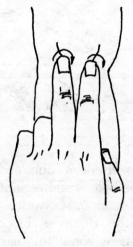

Fig. 3-37 Kneading Guiyan

Therapeutic actions Relieve fright and alleviate pain; tranquilize the Mind.

Indications Acute or chronic infantile convulsion, spasm; flaccidity of the lower limbs.

Kneading Jiexi (Rou Jiexi ST 41)

Site On the dorsum of the foot at the midpoint of the transverse crease of the ankle joint in the depression.

Procedure Knead the point with the thumb or the tip

of the middle finger 30 to 50 times (see Fig. 3-38).

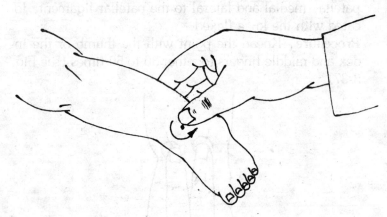

Fig. 3-38   Kneading Jiexi

Therapeutic actions   Relieve fright and tranquilize the Mind; strengthen the Spleen and regulate the Stomach; relieve diarrhea and relax the bowels.
Indications   Headache, dizziness, bloodshot eyes; distention of the abdomen, vomiting, diarrhea, constipation and spasm.

Rotating the Hip Joint While Rotating the Knee (Yao Kuan Xi Jie)

Site   Hip and knee joints.
Procedure   The infant lies face up with the hip and knee flexed. Place one hand on the flexed knee, and hold the ankle with the other, lifting and rotating both knee and hip joints (see Fig. 3-39, 40). Repeat the motion 10 to 20 times.
Therapeutic actions   Promote the circulation of Qi and

76

Blood, relax the tendons and loosen the joints.

Indications Flaccidity of the lower limbs and listlessness.

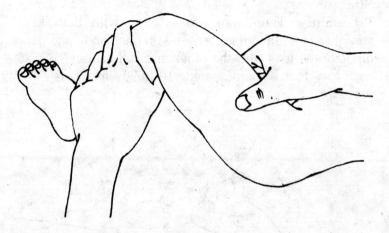

Fig. 3-39 Rotating the hip joint while rotating the knee

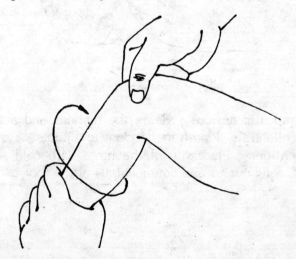

Fig. 3-40 Rotating the hip joint while rotating the knee

77

Pulling and Shaking the Ankle (Yao Huai Jie)

Site Ankle.

Procedure The infant lies face up with both legs straight. Hold the infant's heel with one hand, and manipulate the toes with the other in all directions, rotate each toe, then shake the ankle 10 to 20 times (see Fig. 3-41).

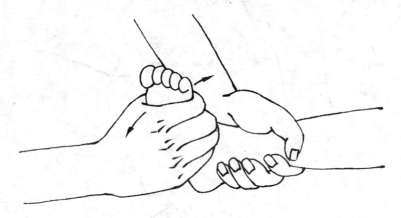

Fig. 3-41 Pulling and shaking the ankle

Therapeutic actions Relax the tendons and activate the collaterals, loosen the tendons and joints.

Indications Flaccidity of the limbs with cold sensation, equinovarus and equinovalgus of the foot.

The Upper Limbs

Kneading Jianyu (Rou Jianyu LI 15)

Site Anterior and inferior to the acromion, in the depression appearing at the anterior border of the acromioclavicular joint.

Procedure Knead the point with the thumb 10 to 20 times (see Fig. 3-42).

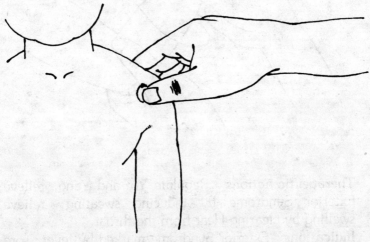

Fig. 3-42 Kneading Jianyu

Therapeutic actions Clear the channels and activate the collaterals; expel Wind and purge Heat.

Indications Rubella due to Wind Heat, paralysis or flaccidity of the arm and shoulder.

Kneading Quchi (Rou Quchi LI 11)

Site In the depression at the lateral end of the transverse cubital crease when the elbow is flexed.

Procedure Hold the wrist with one hand, support the flexed elbow with the other, and then knead the point with the thumb 20 to 30 times (see Fig. 3-43).

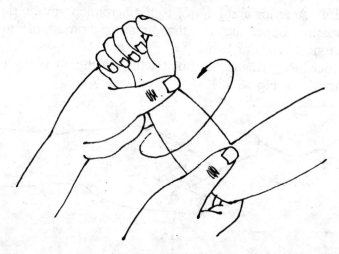

Fig. 3-43 Kneading Quchi

Therapeutic actions Regulate Yin and Yang, relieve Exterior Syndrome by inducing sweating; relieve swelling by clearing Heat from the throat.

Indications Exterior Syndrome marked by fever, sore throat, bloodshot eyes, abdominal pain, vomiting, diarrhea and dysentery.

Grasping Lieque (Na Lieque LU 7)

Site Superior to the styloid process of the radius.
Procedure Place the thumb and index finger lateral to the point, then grasp while pinching 3 to 5 times (see Fig. 3-44).

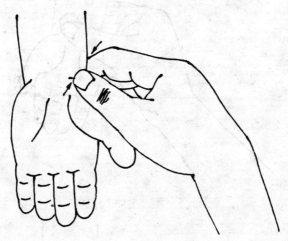

Fig. 3-44 Grasping Lieque

Therapeutic actions Relieve Exterior Syndrome by inducing sweating; stop cough by promoting Lung Qi.
Indications Common cold, headache, stiff neck, cough and asthma.

Kneading Neiguan and Waiguan (Rou Neiguan PC 6 and Waiguan SJ 5)

Site Neiguan is located at the point 2 cun above the transverse crease of the wrist between the two main tendons. Waiguan is located on the outer forearm opposite to Neiguan.

Procedure   Hold the two points with the thumb and index finger in opposition, then knead while pressing 20 to 30 times (see Fig. 3-45, 46, 47).

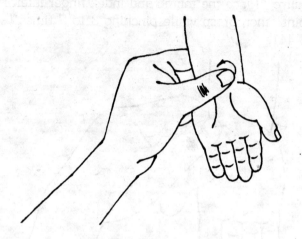

Fig. 3-45   Kneading Neiguan.

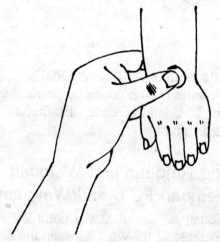

Fig. 3-46   Kneading Waiguan

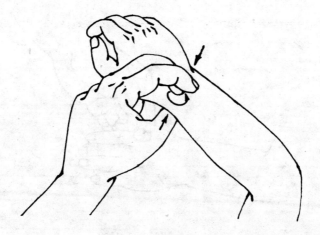

Fig. 3-47 Kneading Neiguan and Waiguan

Therapeutic actions Calm the Heart and tranquilize the Mind; expel Wind and relieve Exterior Syndrome; mediate the Middle Jiao and regulate Stomach Qi.
Indications Common cold, headache, palpitation, insomnia, pain in the upper abdomen and vomiting.

Kneading Hegu (Rou Hegu LI 4)

Site On the dorsal surface of the hand between the first and second metacarpals at the midpoint of the radial side of the second metacarpal.
Procedure Knead with the thumb or middle finger 20 to 30 times (see Fig. 3-48).
Therapeutic actions Relieve Exterior Syndrome by inducing sweating; alleviate pain by clearing Heat; remove lumps by promoting the circulation of Blood and flow of Qi.

83

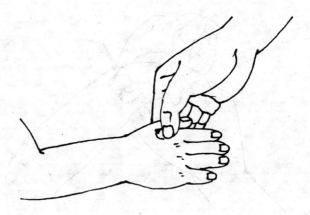

Fig. 3-48   Kneading Hegu

Indications   Headache with stiff neck, fever with no sweats, sore throat, nasal bleeding, toothache, lockjaw, deviation of the mouth and eyes, rebellious Stomach Qi marked by constipation, nausea and vomiting.

Piston Rubbing the Upper Limbs (Cuo Shang Zhi)

Site   The upper limbs.

Procedure   Use both hands to hold the upper limb and friction rub in opposite directions. This motion is repeated from the armpit to the wrist 3 to 5 times (see Fig. 3-49).

Therapeutic actions   Clear the channels and activate the collaterals; promote the flow of Qi and Blood; relax the tendons and loosen the joints.

Indications   Disorders of the shoulder, arm and wrist.

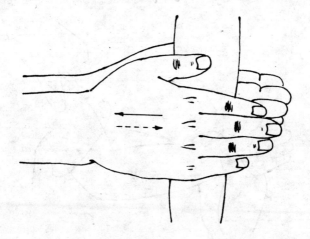

Fig. 3-49 Piston rubbing the upper limb

Rotating and Shaking the Arm (Yao Dou Bi)

Site The upper limb.

Procedure Hold the infant's hand with one hand, and support his shoulder with the other, rotate the arm within a small range while shaking rapidly 5 to 10 times. Finally, support his wrist with one hand, hold his fingers with other, rotate the elbow, wrist and each finger in turn (see Fig. 3-50,51,52,53).

Therapeutic actions Regulate Yin and Yang; clear the Heart and tranquilize the Mind; open the orifices and promote Qi and Blood; relax the tendons and loosen the joints.

Indications Restlessness, night crying due to fright, headache, fever, listlessness, flaccidity and coldness of limbs.

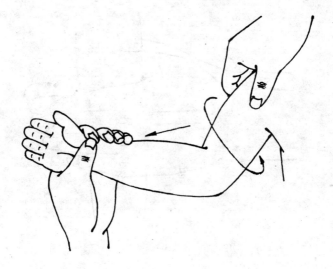

Fig. 3-50   Rotating and shaking the arm

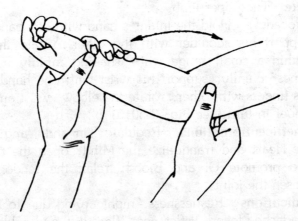

Fig. 3-51   Rotating and shaking the elbow

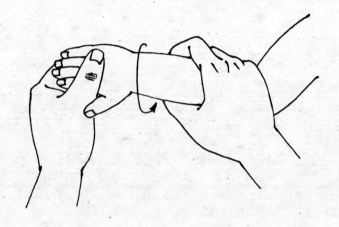

Fig. 3-52   Rotating and shaking the wrist

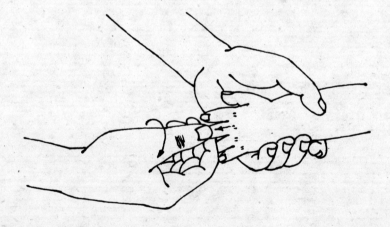

Fig. 3-53   Rotating and regulating the fingers

TREATMENTS USING HAND POINTS AND AREAS

Treatments for Strengthening Body Resistance

Checking Liver Channel (Ping Ganjing)

Site   On the pad of the distal segment of the index finger.

Procedure   Using the thumb, push Liver point toward the fingertip 100 to 500 times (see Fig. 4-1).

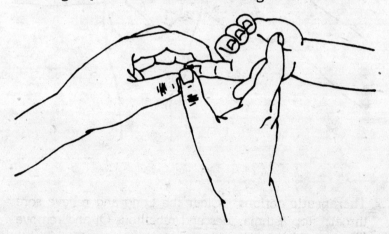

Fig. 4-1   Checking Liver Channel

Therapeutic actions   Soothe depression and relieve irritability; check the Liver and disperse Wind; reduce fever and relax spasm; regulate the flow of Qi and promote the circulation of Blood.

Indications Convulsion with spasms, irritability, crying due to fright, headache, dizziness, five palm heat, bloodshot eyes, dry throat, diarrhea and distention of the abdomen.

Clearing Lung Channel (Qing Feijing)

Site On the pad of the distal segment of the fourth finger.

Procedure Using the thumb, push Lung Channel toward the fingertip 100 to 500 times (see Fig. 4-2).

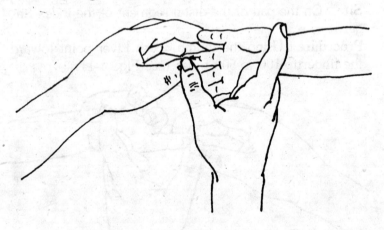

Fig. 4-2 Clearing Lung Channel

Therapeutic actions Clear the Lung and relieve sore throat; stop asthma, descend rebellious Qi and remove Phlegm; relax the bowels.

Indications Common cold marked by fever, cough and asthma with sputum, oppression of the chest, dry

92

stools, dry throat and nose.

Pushing up the Galaxy (Qing Tianheshui)

Site A line from Daling (PC 7) to Quze (PC 3). The midpoint of the forearm between the transverse cubital crease and transverse carpal crease.

Procedure Hold the infant's hand with one hand, push with the index and middle fingers of the other hand from Daling to Quze 100 to 300 times (see Fig. 4-3).

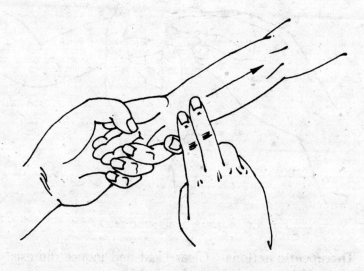

Fig. 4-3 Pushing up the Galaxy

Therapeutic actions Purge Fire and relieve irritability; clear Heat and treat Exterior Syndrome; remove Phlegm and relieve convulsion.

Indications Exterior Syndrome marked by high fever or tidal fever, irritability, night crying due to fright, thirst with desire for cold drinks, numbness of the

93

tongue, sores in mouth, licking the lips, dry bowels and dark urine.

Clearing Small Intestine Channel (Qing Xiaochangjing)

Site   On the ulnar surface of the little finger.

Procedure   Hold the child's hand with one hand, push with the thumb of the other hand toward the fingertip 100 to 300 times (see Fig. 4-4).

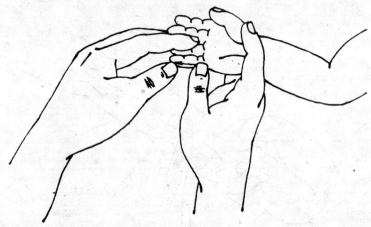

Fig. 4-4   Clearing Small Intestine Channel

Therapeutic actions   Clear Heat and induce diuresis; lift lucid Yang and descend turbid Yin.

Indications   Dark urine with painful urination, and even retention of urine, sores in the mouth, or watery stools.

Kneading Xiaotianxin (Rou Xiaotianxin)

Site   In the depression between the two thenar emi-

94

nences at the base of the palm.

Procedure Hold the infant's hand with the palm up and knead the point with the index or middle finger of the other hand 50 to 300 times (see Fig. 4-5).

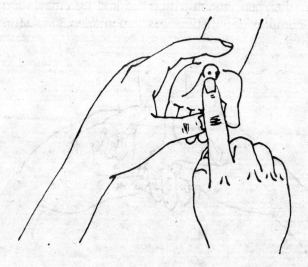

Fig. 4-5 Kneading Xiaotianxin

Therapeutic actions Clear Heart Fire; induce diuresis; tranquilize the Mind and relieve fright; open the orifices and disperse accumulation; improve vision.

Indications Convulsion with spasm, irritability, dark urine, night crying, or measles with partial eruptions.

Reinforcing Spleen Channel (Bu Pijing)

Site The ulnar edge of the thumb.

Procedure Hold one hand of the infant, push the area toward the thumb tip with the practitioner's thumb 200 to 500 times (see Fig. 4-6).

Therapeutic actions Strengthen the Spleen and regu-

95

late the Stomach; tonify Qi and nourish Blood; remove food stagnation and promote digestion; clear Phlegm and improve appetite.

Indications Loss of appetite, distention of the abdomen, diarrhea, malnutrition marked by emaciation, dusky complexion, listlessness, spontaneous sweating or night sweats.

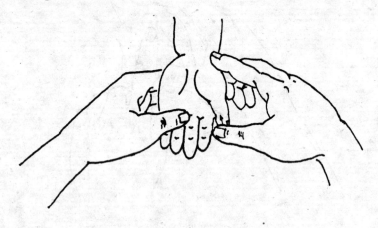

Fig. 4-6 Reinforcing Spleen Channel

Reinforcing Kidney Channel (Bu Shenjing)

Site On the pad of distal segment of little finger.

Procedure Knead with the thumb from the fingertip toward the palm 100 to 500 times (see Fig. 4-7).

Therapeutic actions Reinforce the Kidney and benefit the brain; tonify Qi and clear the Mind; relieve asthma by leading Qi toward the Kidney; warm Kidney Yang and clear Deficiency Fire.

Indications Weakness, diarrhea before dawn, bed-wetting, frequent urination, cough, shortness of

96

breath, toothache due to rising of Deficiency Fire, five kinds of retardation and flaccidity.

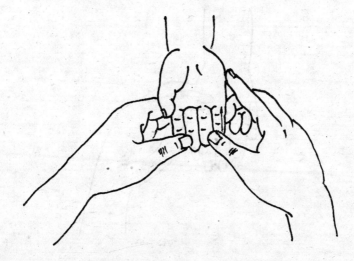

Fig. 4-7   Reinforcing Kidney Channel

Kneading Errenshangma (Rou Errenshangma)

Site   On the dorsum of the hand, in the depression between the distal ends of the fourth and fifth metacarpals.

Procedure   Knead the point with the thumb or middle finger 100 to 300 times (see Fig. 4-8).

Therapeutic actions   Nourish the Kidney and suppress Yang; lead Fire back to the Kidney; disperse accumulation by promoting the flow of Qi.

Indications   Painful urination with discomfort, dark urine, swelling and pain of the throat, unconsciousness, tinnitus, mild fever, pain of the abdomen and flaccidity of the lower limbs.

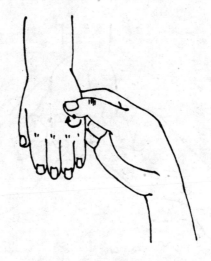

Fig. 4-8 Kneading Errenshangma

Kneading Banmen (Rou Banmen)

Site   The midpoint of the thenar eminence.

Procedure   Knead with the thumb or middle finger 50 to 300 times (see Fig. 4-9).

Therapeutic actions - Strengthen the Spleen and regulate the Stomach; remove food stagnation and disperse accumulation; relieve distention and stop vomiting.

Indications   Loss of appetite, food retained in the stomach, nausea, vomiting, diarrhea, distention of the abdomen, belching and foul breath.

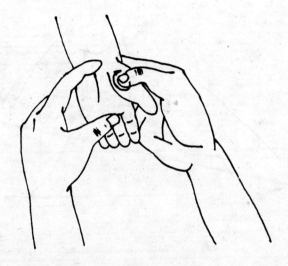

Fig. 4-9 Kneading Banmen

Clearing and Reinforcing
the Large Intestine Channel
(Qing Bu Dachangjing)

Site On the radial surface of the index finger.

Procedure Hold the other fingers and push with the thumb 100 to 300 times (see Fig. 4-10). Push toward the hand to reinforce, away from the hand to clear.

Therapeutic actions Clear the Large Intestine, remove Damp Heat and accumulation; reinforce the Large Intestine, stop diarrhea and warm the Middle Jiao.

Indications Pain and fullness of the abdomen, dysentery due to Damp Heat, diarrhea due to Heat, prolapse of the anus, redness and swelling around the anus, cough due to Lung Heat.

99

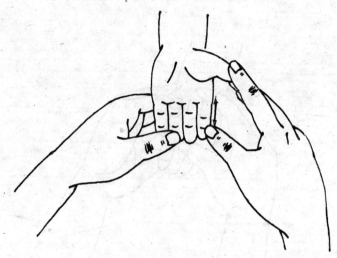

Fig. 4-10   Clearing and reinforcing the
Large Intestine Channel

100

Treatments
for Preventing
Respiratory Disorders

Clearing Lung Channel
(Qing Feijing)
See Page 92 and Fig. 4-11.

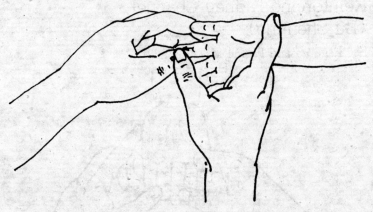

Fig. 4-11   Clearing Lung Channel

Reinforcing Spleen
Channel (Bu Pijing)
See Page 95 and Fig. 4-12.

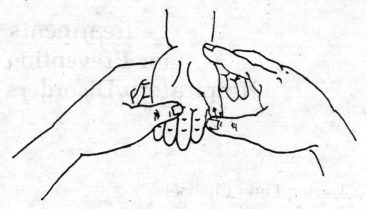

Fig. 4-12   Reinforcing Spleen Channel

Reinforcing Kidney Channel
(Bu Shenjing)

See Page 96 and Fig. 4-13.

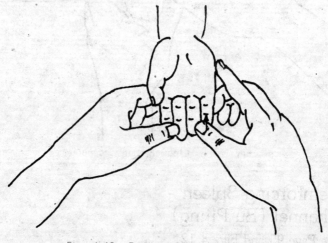

Fig. 4-13   Reinforcing Kidney Channel

Kneading Errenshangma
(Rou Errenshangma)

See Page 97 and Fig. 4-14.

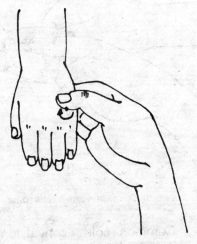

Fig. 4-14 Kneading Errenshangma

General therapeutic actions   Tonify and restore Lung Qi, prevent and treat common cold.

Kneading Yiwofeng (Rou Yiwofeng)

Site   On the dorsum of the hand, midway between Yangxi (LI 5) and Yangchi (SJ 4), in the depression when the hand is extended.

Procedure   Hold the hand with one hand, and knead the point with the thumb or middle finger of the other 100 to 300 times (see Fig. 4-15).

Therapeutic actions   Expel Wind and disperse Cold; warm the Middle Jiao and regulate the flow of Qi; relieve fright and tranquilize the Mind; alleviate pain.

103

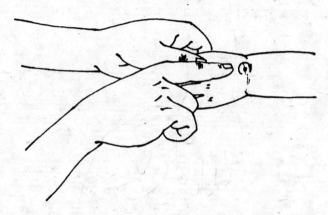

Fig. 4-15 Kneading Yiwofeng

Indications Common cold, convulsion, headache, fullness of the chest and distention of the abdomen.

Kneading Ershanmen (Rou Ershanmen)

Site On the dorsal surface of the hand on both sides of the metacarpophalangeal joint of the middle finger.

Procedure Knead the points with the index and middle fingers simultaneously 100 to 300 times (see Fig. 4-16).

Therapeutic actions Relieve Exterior Syndrome; reduce fever and stop cough; expel Wind and activate collaterals.

Indications Common cold, fever without sweating, convulsion with spasm, deviation of the eyes and mouth.

104

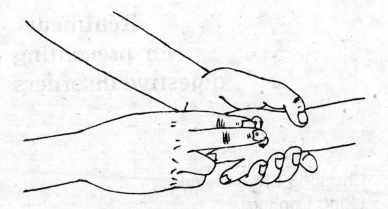

Fig. 4-16   Kneading Ershanmen

Treatments for preventing digestive disorders

Checking Liver Channel (Ping Ganjing)

See Page 91 and Fig. 4-17.

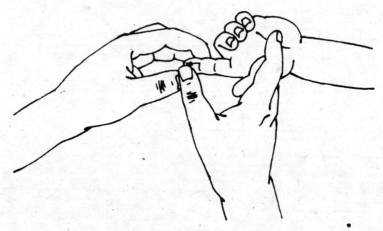

Fig. 4-17 Checking Liver Channel

Reinforcing Spleen Channel (Bu Pijing)

See Page 95 and Fig. 4-18.

106

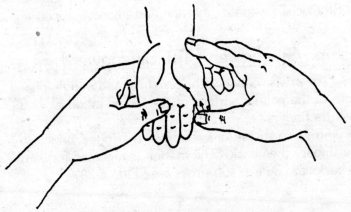

Fig. 4-18 Reinforcing Spleen Channel

Kneading Banmen (Rou Banmen)

See Page 98 and Fig. 4-19.

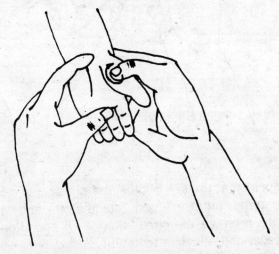

Fig. 4-19 Kneading Banmen

General therapeutic actions Strengthen the Spleen and Stomach, promote digestion and improve appetite.

Pushing Sihengwen (Tui Sihengwen)

Site The crease between the proximal and middle phalanges of the palmar surface of the index, middle, ring and little fingers.

Procedure Push the creases from the index finger to little finger, then back. The motion is repeated forward and backward 300 to 400 times (see Fig. 4-20).

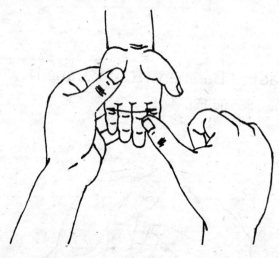

Fig. 4-20 Pushing Sihengwen

Therapeutic actions Soothe the chest and relax the diaphragm; remove food stagnation and resolve Phlegm; promote the circulation of Qi and Blood; reduce fever and alleviate irritability.

Indications Pain and distention of the abdomen, malnutrition, loss of appetite, asthma with mucus accumu-

108

lation, sores in the mouth and lips.

Circular Gliding Bagua (Yun Bagua)

Site A circle with Laogong (PC 8) at the center.
Procedure Hold four fingers with one hand, and glide with the thumb of the other in a circular motion 50 to 200 times (see Fig. 4-21).

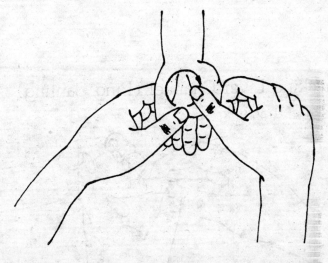

Fig. 4-21 Circular gliding Bagua

Therapeutic actions Soothe the chest and regulate the flow of Qi; remove food stagnation and disperse accumulation; resolve Phlegm and relieve cough.
Indications Fullness of the chest and distention of the abdomen, loss of appetite, vomiting, diarrhea, or irritability, or cough.

Treatments
for Preventing
Nervous Disorders

Checking Liver Channel (Ping Ganjing)

See Page 91 and Fig. 4-22.

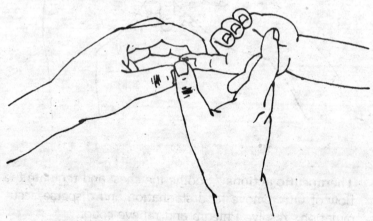

Fig. 4-22   Checking Liver Channel

Kneading Xiaotianxin
(Rou Xiaotianxin)

See Page 94 and Fig. 4-23.

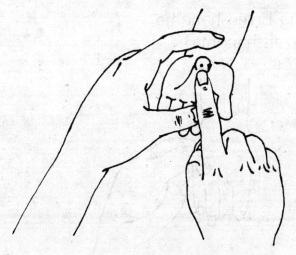

Fig. 4-23   Kneading Xiaotianxin

Reinforcing Kidney Channel
(Bu Shenjing)

See Page 96 and Fig. 4-24.

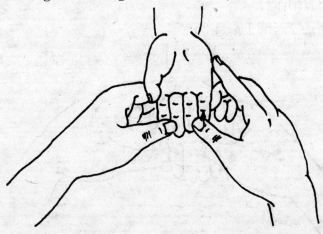

Fig. 4-24   Reinforcing Kidney Channel

111

Kneading Errenshangma
(Rou Errenshangma)
See Page 97 Fig. 4-25.

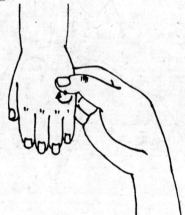

Fig. 4-25   Kneading Errenshangma

Reinforcing Spleen Channel
(Bu Pijing)
See Page 95 and Fig. 4-26.

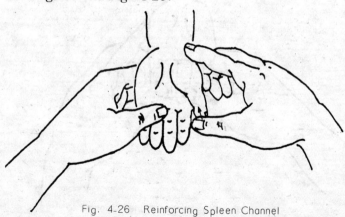

Fig. 4-26   Reinforcing Spleen Channel

112

Clearing Small Intestine Channel
(Qing Xiaochangjing)

See Page 94 and Fig. 4-27.

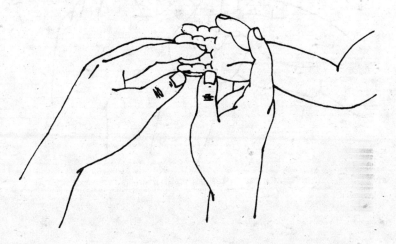

Fig. 4-27 Clearing Small Intestine Channel

General therapeutic actions Strengthen the brain and benefit mentality; relieve fright and tranquilize the Mind.

Clearing Heart Channel
(Qing Xinjing)

Site The pad of the distal segment of the middle finger.

Procedure Push with the thumb toward the fingertip 100 to 300 times (see Fig. 4-28).

Therapeutic actions Clear Heart Fire; tonify Qi and Blood; nourish the Heart and tranquilize the Mind.

Indications High fever, five palm heat, irritability,

113

sores in the mouth, dark urine, oppression of the chest, palpitation due to Deficiency of Heart Blood.

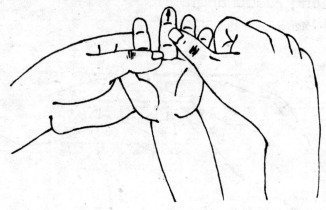

Fig. 4-28   Clearing Heart Channel

Treatments
for Preventing
Urinary Disorders

Reinforcing Kidney Channel
(Bu Shenjing)

See Page 96 and Fig. 4-29.

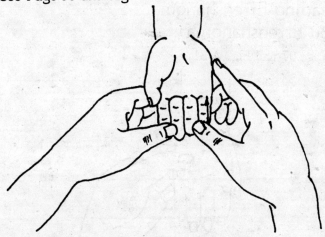

Fig. 4-29   Reinforcing Kidney Channel

Reinforcing Spleen Channel
(Bu Pijing)

See Page 95 and Fig. 4-30.

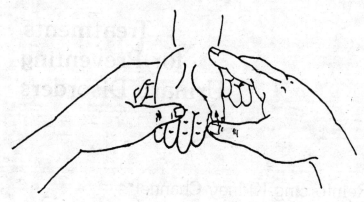

Fig. 4-30   Reinforcing Spleen Channel

Kneading Errenshangma
(Rou Errenshangma)

See Page 97 and Fig. 4-31.

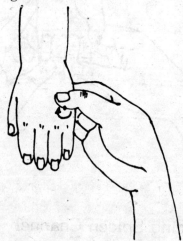

Fig. 4-31   Kneading Errenshangma

116

General therapeutic actions Reinforce the Kidney and tonify Qi; relax the bowels and consolidate Kidney Yang.

Pushing Sanguan (Tui Sanguan)

Site The line from the wrist crease along the radial surface of the forearm to Quchi (LI 11).
Procedure With the index and middle fingers together, push along this line from the wrist to the elbow 100 to 300 times (see Fig. 4-32).

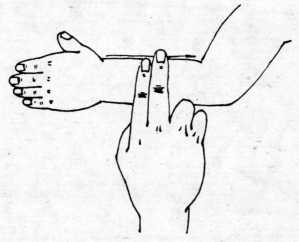

Fig. 4-32   Pushing Sanguan

Therapeutic actions Tonify Qi and nourish Blood; reinforce Kidney Qi and reduce weakness; warm Yang and disperse Cold.
Indications Anemia, weakness and coldness of limbs, spontaneous sweating, or bed-wetting.

117

TREATMENT
FOR COMMONLY
ENCOUNTERED
DISORDERS

Common Cold

Common cold is identified as an Exterior Syndrome in TCM. It may occur in any season, but particularly in winter and spring.

Etiology and Pathogenesis

Zangfu Organs in infants are not completely developed and Defensive Qi is not yet strong enough to counter an invasion of external pathogenic factors. Therefore, the common cold may occur if Wind Cold or Wind Heat attacks the Exterior of the body.

Treatment Based on Syndrome Identification

Common cold due to Wind Cold

Manifestations   Mild fever, or no fever or sweating, chills, headache, stuffy or running nose with thin discharge, cough with a little sputum. Red tongue with thin white coating, floating red superficial venule of the index finger.

Treatment principle   Relieve Exterior Syndrome by inducing sweating.

Prescription   Opening Tianmen (see Fig. 5-1), Pushing Kangong (see Fig. 5-2), circular gliding Taiyang (see Fig 5-3), circular gliding Erhougaogu (see Fig. 5-4), pushing Sanguan (see Fig. 5-5), clearing and reinforcing Spleen Channel (see Fig. 5-6), kneading Yiwofeng (see Fig. 5-7), kneading Ershanmen (see Fig.

121

5-8) and kneading Feishu (BL 13) (see Fig. 5-9).
Medium   Chinese onion juice or ginger juice.

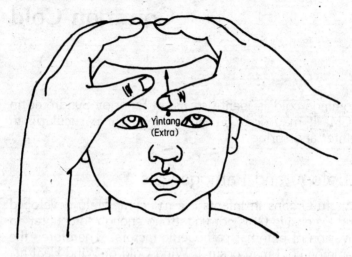

Fig. 5-1   Opening Tianmen

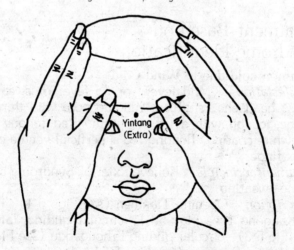

Fig. 5-2   Pushing Kangong

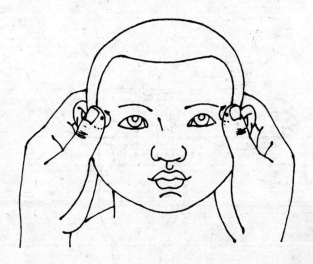

Fig. 5-3   Circular gliding Taiyang

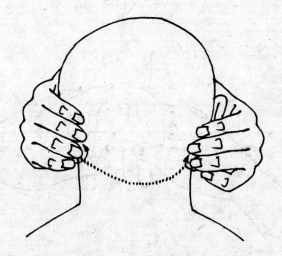

Fig. 5-4   Circular gliding Erhougaogu

123

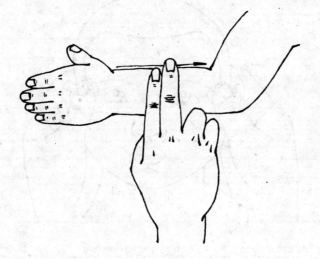

Fig. 5-5   Pushing Sanguan

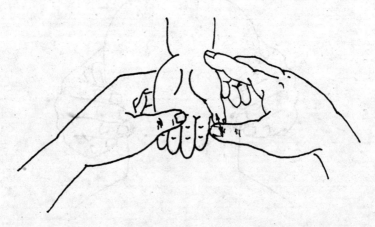

Fig. 5-6   Clearing and reinforcing Spleen Channel

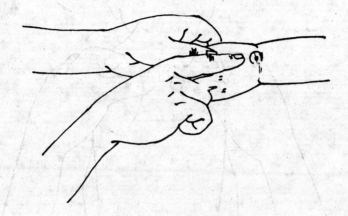

Fig. 5-7   Kneading Yiwofeng

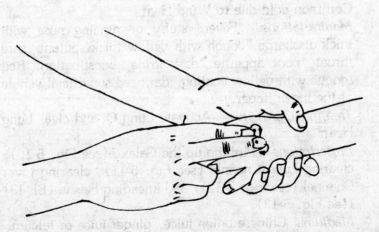

Fig. 5-8   Kneading Ershanmen

125

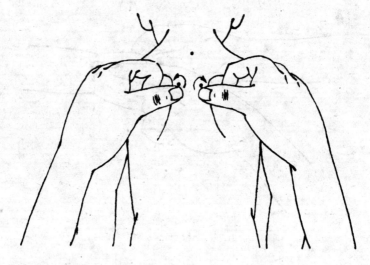

Fig. 5-9 Kneading Feishu

Common cold due to Wind Heat
Manifestations   Fever, stuffy or running nose with thick discharge, cough with yellow thick sputum, sore throat, poor appetite, dark urine, constipation. Red tongue with yellow coating, dark red superficial venule of the index finger.

Treatment principle   Activate Lung Qi and clear Lung Heat.

Prescriptions   Pushing up the Galaxy (see Fig. 5-10), clearing Lung Channel (see Fig. 5-11), clearing Liver Channel (see Fig. 5-12), and kneading Feishu (BL 13) (see Fig. 5-13).

Medium   Chinese onion juice, ginger juice or talcum.

126

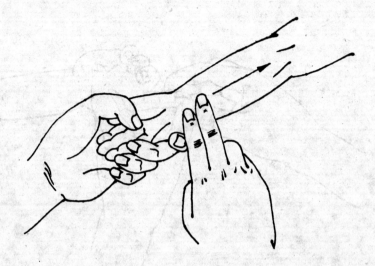

Fig. 5-10   Pushing up the Galaxy

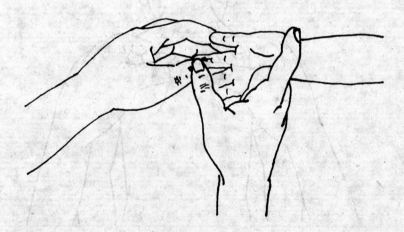

Fig. 5-11   Clearing Lung Channel

127

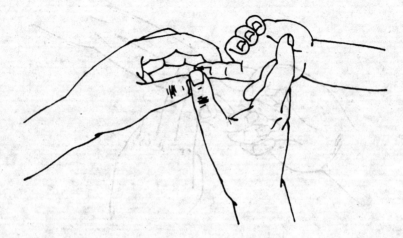

Fig. 5-12   Clearing Liver Channel

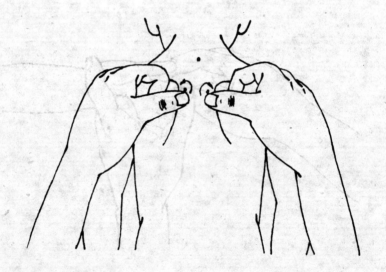

Fig. 5-13   Kneading Feishu

128

Diarrhea

Infant diarrhea more often occurs in summer time and autumn.

Etiology and Pathogenesis

The function of the Spleen and Stomach in infants is not completely developed, so diarrhea may occur either because of the invasion of external pathogens or due to dysfunction of internal Zangfu Organs.

Treatment Based on Syndrome Identification

Diarrhea due to Damp Heat

Manifestations　Diarrhea with yellow, thin or watery stools with foul odor, painful abdomen, irritability, thirst, redness, swelling and burning sensation around the anus, dark urine, oliguria. Yellow greasy tongue coating, purple superficial venule of the index finger.

Treatment principle　Clear Heat and remove Damp; regulate the Middle Jiao and stop diarrhea.

Prescription　Clearing and reinforcing Spleen Channel (see Fig. 5-14), clearing Stomach Channel (see Fig. 5-15), clearing Large Intestine Channel (see Fig. 5-16), clearing Small Intestine Channel (See Fig. 5-17), kneading Guiwei (see Fig. 5-18) and pressing and kneading Zusanli (ST 36) (see Fig. 5-19).

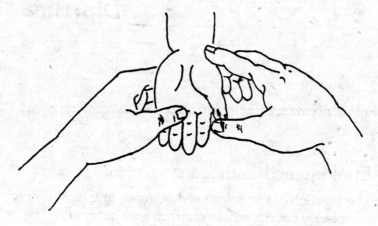

Fig. 5-14 Clearing and reinforcing Spleen Channel

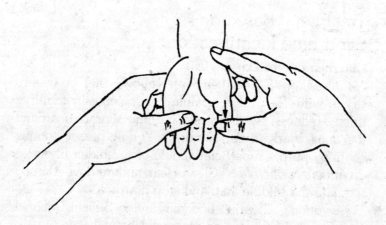

Fig. 5-15 Clearing Stomach Channel

130

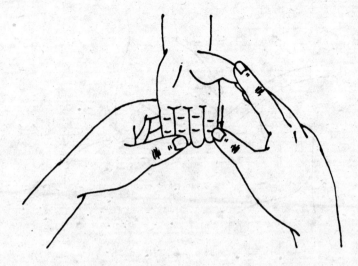

Fig. 5-16 Clearing Large Intestine Channel

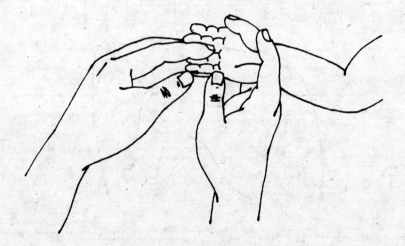

Fig. 5-17 Clearing Small Intestine Channel

131

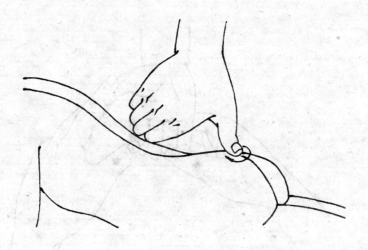

Fig. 5-18   Kneading Guiwei

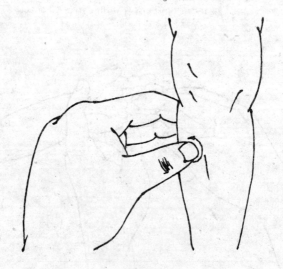

Fig. 5-19   Pressing and kneading Zusanli

Medium   Talcum or cold water.
Diarrhea due to Cold Damp

Manifestations   Diarrhea with thin, frothy stools, painful abdomen with desire for warmth and pressure, bowel sounds, lack of thirst, aversion to cold, cold limbs, poor appetite. Pale tongue with white greasy coating, light red superficial venule of the index finger.

Treatment principle   Warm the Middle Jiao to disperse Cold; remove Damp to relieve diarrhea.

Prescription   Pushing Sanguan (see Fig. 5-20), kneading Yiwofeng (see Fig. 5-21), reinforcing Spleen Channel (see Fig. 5-22), reinforcing Large Intestine Channel (see Fig. 5-23), circular rubbing Shenque (REN 8) (see Fig. 5-24), kneading Guiwei (see Fig. 5-25) and pushing up Qijiegu (see Fig. 5-26).

Medium   Talcum, Chinese onion juice or ginger juice.

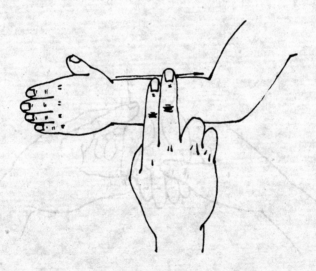

Fig. 5-20   Pushing Sanguan

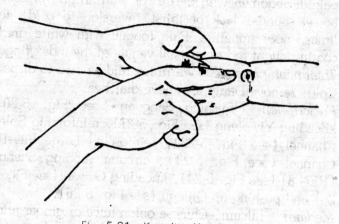

Fig. 5-21 Kneading Yiwofeng

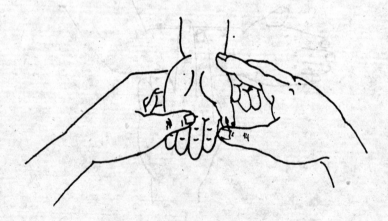

Fig. 5-22 Reinforcing Spleen Channel

134

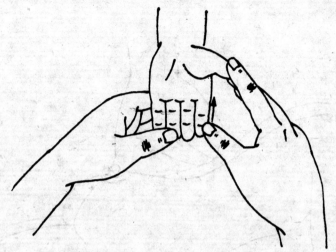

Fig. 5-23   Reinforcing Large Intestine Channel

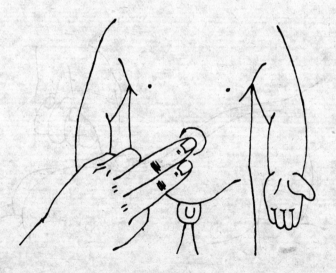

Fig. 5-24   Circular rubbing Shenque

135

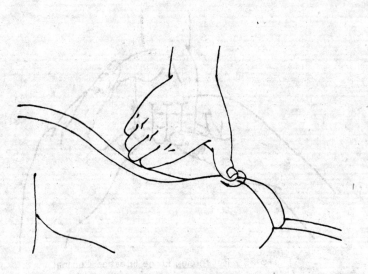

Fig. 5-25 Kneading Guiwei

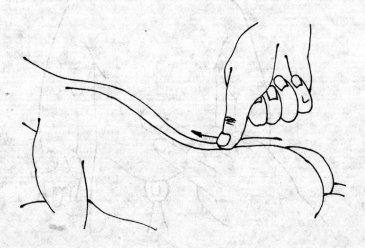

Fig. 5-26 Pushing up Qijiegu

136

Diarrhea due to food stagnation

Manifestations　Diarrhea with thin foul stools, distention and fullness of the abdomen aggravated by pressure, hiccups, acid regurgitation, pain in the abdomen relieved by defecation, loss of appetite, or vomiting. Thick greasy tongue coating, dim purple superficial venule of the index finger.

Treatment principle　Remove food stagnation and disperse accumulation; regulate the Middle Jiao and strengthen the Stomach.

Prescription　Clearing and reinforcing Spleen Channel (see Fig. 5-27), clearing Large Intestine Channel (see Fig. 5-28), kneading Banmen (see Fig. 5-29), separating Yin and Yang of the abdomen (see Fig. 5-30), pushing Sihengwen (see Fig. 5-31) and circular gliding Bagua (see Fig. 5-32).

Medium　Talcum.

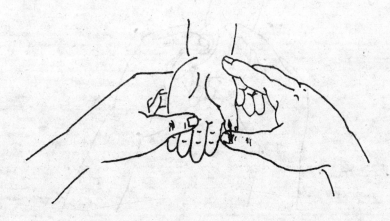

Fig. 5-27　Clearing and reinforcing Spleen Channel

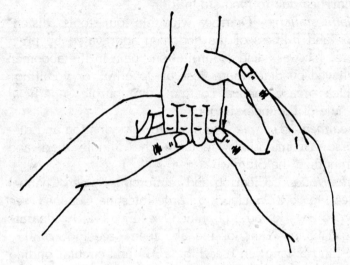

Fig. 5-28   Clearing Large Intestine Channel

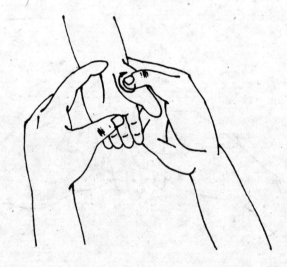

Fig. 5-29   Kneading Banmen

138

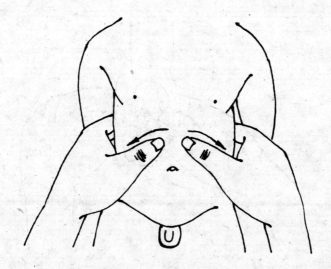

Fig. 5-30　Separating Yin and Yang of the abdomen

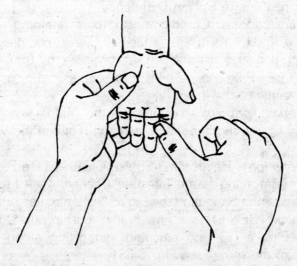

Fig. 5-31　Pushing Sihengwen

139

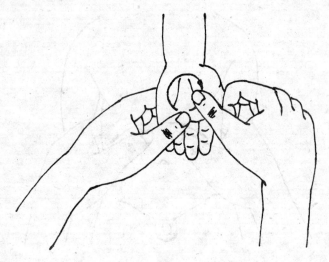

Fig. 5-32   Circular gliding Bagua

Diarrhea due to Spleen Deficiency

Manifestations   Chronic loose stools retaining undi-
gested food, recurrent attacks, dusky complexion,
emaciation and listlessness; or prolapse of the anus,
pale face. Pale tongue with thin coating, pale superficial venule of the index finger.

Treatment principle   Reinforce the Middle Jiao and
tonify Qi; strengthen the Spleen and regulate the Stomach.

Prescription   Reinforcing Spleen Channel (see Fig. 5-
33), reinforcing Large Intestine Channel (see Fig. 5-
34), pushing Sanguan (see Fig. 5-35), circular rubbing
Shenque (REN 8) (see Fig. 5-36), pushing up Qijiegu
(see Fig. 5-37) and pinching and lifting along both
sides of the spine (see Fig. 5-38).

Medium   Warm water or talcum.

140

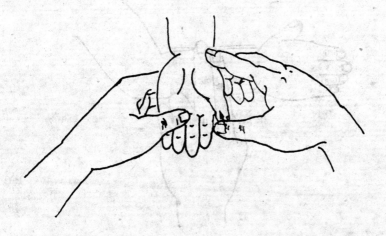

Fig. 5-33 Reinforcing Spleen Channel

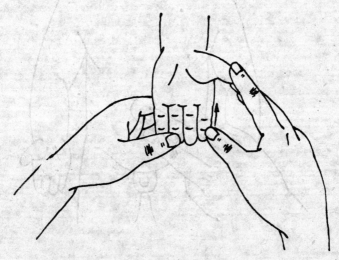

Fig. 5-34 Reinforcing Large Intestine Channel

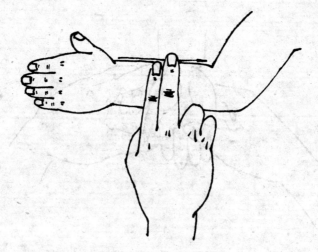

Fig. 5-35 Pushing Sanguan

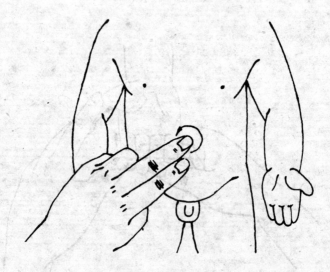

Fig. 5-36 Circular rubbing Shenque

142

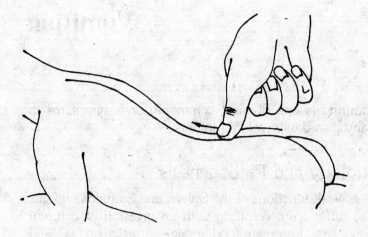

Fig. 5-37   Pushing up Qijiegu

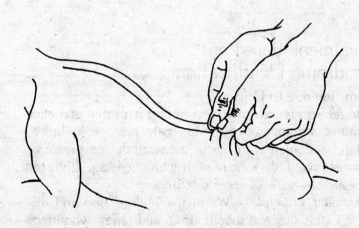

Fig. 5-38   Pinching and lifting along
both sides of the spine

143

Vomiting

Vomiting is one of most commonly seen symptoms in many disorders involving infants.

Etiology and Pathogenesis

With weak functions of the Spleen and Stomach, infants may suffer from vomiting with an invasion of external pathogens, improper food intake, attacks of fear and terror, traumatic injury or Excess Heat-Deficiency Cold of the Spleen and Stomach lead to rebellious Stomach Qi.

Treatment Based on Syndrome Identification

Vomiting due to Cold

Manifestations   Recurrent vomiting with thin and clear vomitus, aggravated by cold, pale face, cold limbs, painful abdomen with desire for warmth and pressure, loose stools. Pale tongue with white coating, light red superficial venule of the index finger.

Treatment principle   Warm the Middle Jiao and disperse Cold; descend rebellious Qi and relieve vomiting.

Prescription   Reinforcing Spleen Channel (see Fig. 5-39), pushing Sanguan (see Fig. 5-40), pushing Sihengwen toward Banmen (see Fig. 5-41) and kneading Zhongwan (REN 12) (see Fig. 5-42).

144

Medium   Ginger juice.

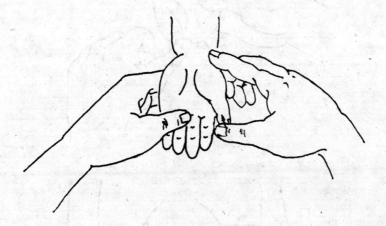

Fig. 5-39   Reinforcing Spleen Channel

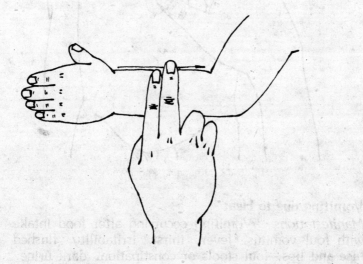

Fig. 5-40   Pushing Sanguan

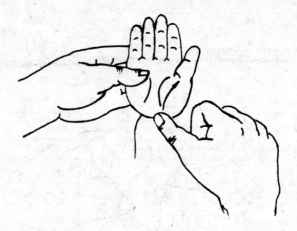

Fig. 5-41 Pushing Sihengwen toward Banmen

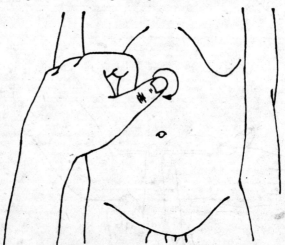

Fig. 5-42 Kneading Zhongwan

Vomiting due to Heat

Manifestations   Vomiting occurring after food intake with foul vomitus, fever, thirst, irritability, flushed face and lips, foul stools or constipation, dark urine. Red tongue with yellow coating, dark or purple superficial venule of the index finger.

Treatment principle   Clear Heat and regulate the

146

Stomach; descend rebellious Qi and relieve vomiting.

Prescription   Clearing Spleen Channel (see Fig. 5-43), clearing Stomach Channel (see Fig. 5-44), kneading Banmen (see Fig. 5-45), circular gliding Bagua (see Fig. 5-46), pushing Xiaohengwen toward Banmen (see Fig. 5-47) and clearing Large Intestine Channel (see Fig. 5-48).

Medium   Cold water or talcum.

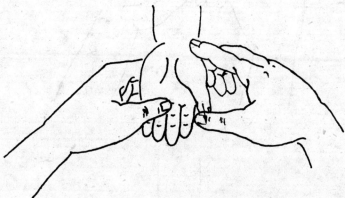

Fig. 5-43   Clearing Spleen Channel

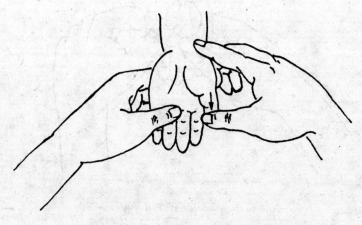

Fig. 5-44   Clearing Stomach Channel

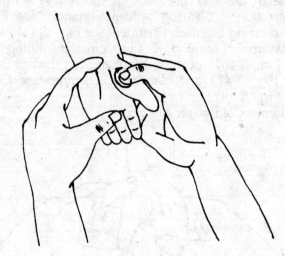

Fig. 5-45 Kneading Banmen

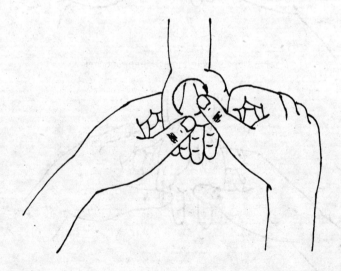

Fig. 5-46 Circular gliding Bagua

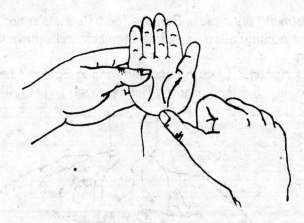

Fig. 5-47　Pushing Xiaohengwen toward Banmen

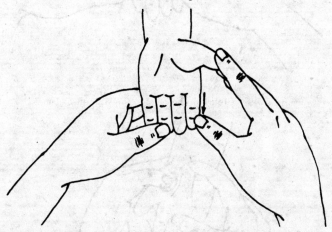

Fig. 5-48　Clearing Large Intestine Channel

Vomiting due to improper food intake

Manifestations　　Fullness and distention of the abdomen, restlessness due to discomfort in the abdomen, acid regurgitation, distaste for food, vomiting with foul odor, foul stools. Thick greasy tongue coating, dark purple superficial venule of the index finger.

Treatment principle   Remove food stagnation and disperse accumulation; regulate Stomach and relieve vomiting.

Prescription   Clearing and reinforcing Spleen Channel (see Fig. 5-49), kneading Banmen (see Fig. 5-50),

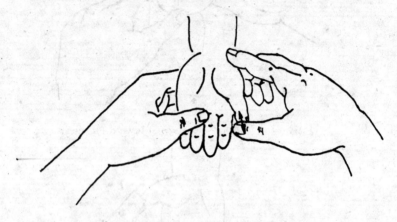

Fig. 5-49   Clearing and reinforcing Spleen Channel

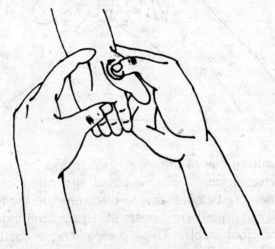

Fig. 5-50   Kneading Banmen

clearing Stomach Channel (see Fig. 5-51), separating Yin and Yang of the abdomen (see Fig. 5-52) and pressing and rubbing down the sides of the body (see Fig. 5-53).
Medium Talcum.

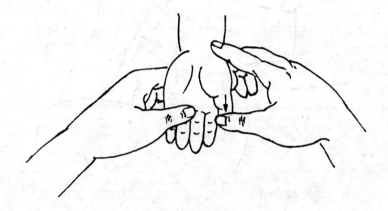

Fig. 5-51   Clearing Stomach Channel

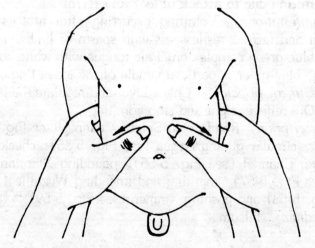

Fig. 5-52   Separating Yin and Yang of abdomen

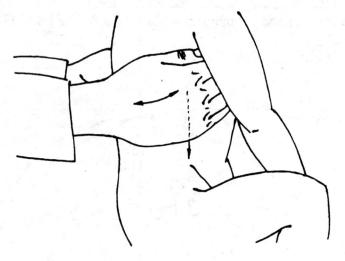

Fig. 5-53 Pressing and rubbing down
the sides of the body

Vomiting due to attack of fear and terror

Manifestations   Vomiting occurring after attacks of
fear and terror, restlessness with spasm of limbs, pale
or blue-green complexion. Pale tongue with white coating, blue-green superficial venule of the index finger.

Treatment principle   Check Liver and regulate the flow
of Qi; relieve fright and stop vomiting.

Prescription   Reinforcing Spleen Channel (see Fig. 5-
54), circular gliding Bagua (see Fig. 5-55), checking
Liver Channel (see Fig. 5-56), pounding Xiaotianxin
(see Fig. 5-57), marking and kneading Wuzhijie (see
Fig. 5-58) and pushing Xinmen (see Fig. 5-59).

Medium   Talcum.

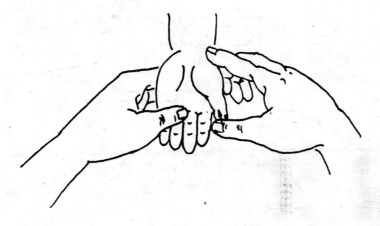

Fig. 5-54   Reinforcing Spleen Channel

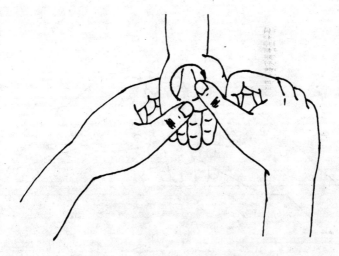

Fig. 5-55   Circular gliding Bagua

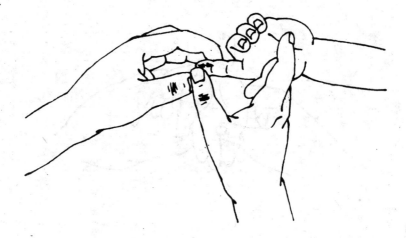

Fig. 5-56   Checking Liver Channel

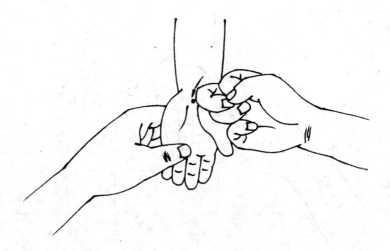

Fig. 5-57   Pounding Xiaotianxin

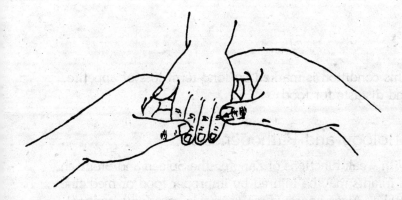

Fig. 5-58 Marking and kneading Wuzhijie

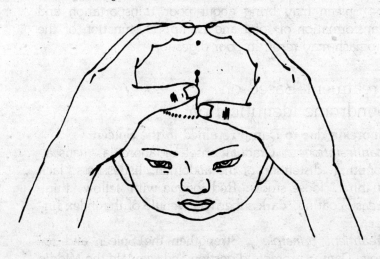

Fig. 5-59 Pushing Xinmen

155

Anorexia

This condition is marked by long-term loss of appetite, and distaste for food.

Etiology and Pathogenesis

With weak functions of Zangfu, the Spleen and Stomach in infants may be injured by improper food or medicine intake. Also, anorexia may occur in cases with congenital weakness of the Spleen and Stomach. Dysfunction of the Spleen may bring about poor transportation and transformation of food and Damp; Dysfunction of the Stomach may result in poor digestion.

Treatment Based on Syndrome Identification

Anorexia due to Damp retained in the Spleen

Manifestations   Gradual onset of anorexia, nausea, vomiting, distention of the abdomen, listlessness, lack of thirst, loose stools. Red tongue with yellow, thin, greasy coating, dark superficial venule of the index finger.

Treatment principle   Strengthen the Spleen and remove Damp; promote digestion and regulate the Middle Jiao.

Prescription   Reinforcing Spleen Channel (see Fig. 5-60), kneading Banmen (see Fig. 5-61), separating Yin and Yang of the abdomen (see Fig. 5-62), pushing Si-hengwen (see Fig. 5-63), kneading Pishu (BL 20) (see Fig. 5-64) and pinching and lifting along both sides of the spine (see Fig. 5-65).

Medium Talcum.

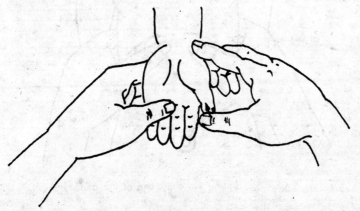

Fig. 5-60   Reinforcing Spleen Channel

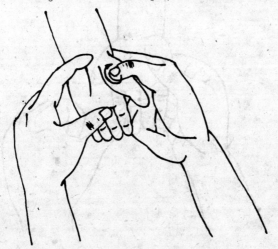

Fig. 5-61   Kneading Banmen

157

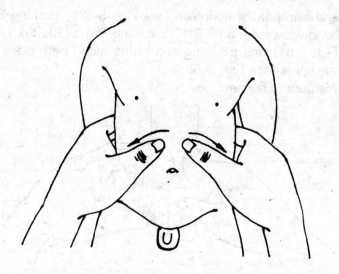

Fig. 5-62   Separating Yin and Yang of the abdomen

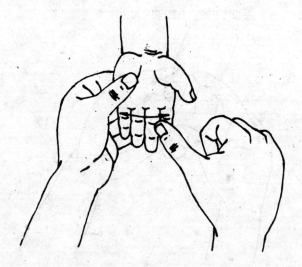

Fig. 5-63   Pushing Sihengwen

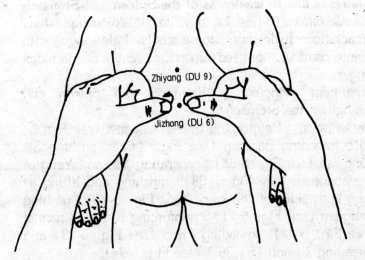

Zhiyang (DU 9)

Jizhong (DU 6)

Fig. 5-64 Kneading Pishu

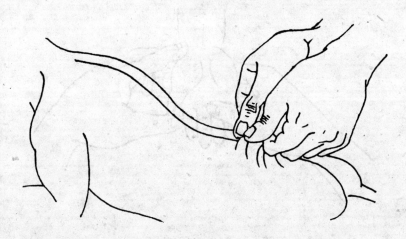

Fig. 5-65 Pinching and lifting along
both sides of the spine

159

Anorexia due to weakness of the Spleen and Stomach

Manifestations   Loss of appetite, dusky complexion, emaciation, listlessness, loose stools. Pale tongue with scanty coating, light red superficial venule of the index finger.

Treatment principle   Reinforce the Spleen and strengthen the Stomach.

Prescription   Reinforcing Spleen Channel (see Fig. 5-66), kneading Banmen (see Fig. 5-67), pushing Sihengwen (see Fig. 5-68), separating Yin and Yang of the abdomen (see Fig. 5-69), pinching and lifting along both sides of the spine (see Fig. 5-70), pushing Sanguan (see Fig. 5-71), reinforcing Kidney Channel (see Fig. 5-72), kneading Erma (see Fig. 5-73) and kneading Zusanli (ST 36) (see Fig. 5-74).

Medium   Talcum.

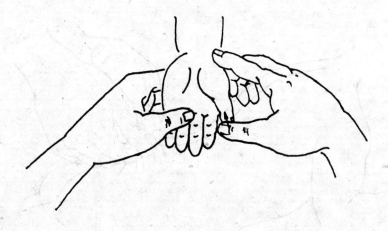

Fig. 5-66   Reinforcing Spleen Channel

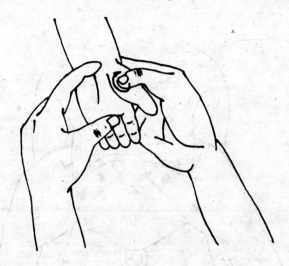

Fig. 5-67   Kneading Banmen

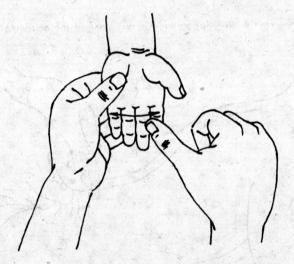

Fig. 5-68   Pushing Sihengwen

161

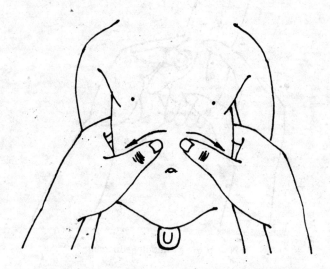

Fig. 5-69   Separating Yin and Yang of the abdomen

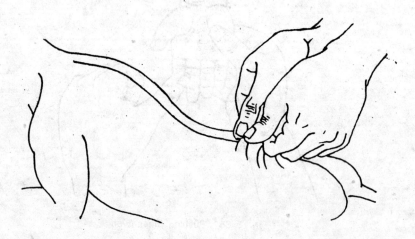

Fig. 5-70   Pinching and lifting along
both sides of the spine

162

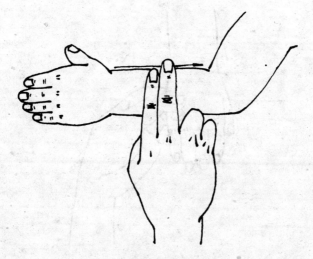

Fig. 5-71   Pushing Sanguan

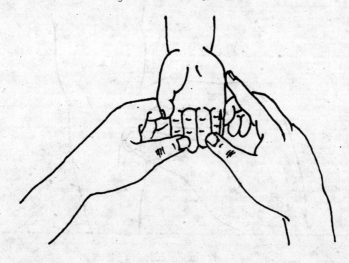

Fig. 5-72   Reinforcing Kidney Channel

163

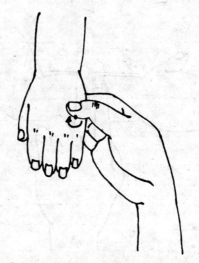

Fig. 5-73 Kneading Erma

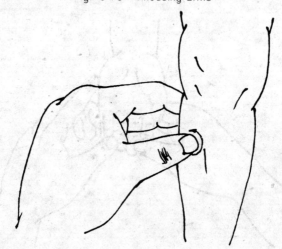

Fig. 5-74 Kneading Zusanli (ST 36)

Constipation

This condition is marked by dry stools with difficult bowel movements, or no bowel movement for several days.

Etiology and Pathogenesis

Congenital weakness may lead to Deficiency of Kidney Yang; improper nursing during illness may result in Deficiency of Blood and Qi; Heat accumulated in the Stomach and Large Intestine may bring about stagnation of Qi, so constipation occurs.

Treatment Based on Syndrome Identification

Constipation seen in Excess Syndrome

Manifestations   Dry stools with no bowel movement for several days, dark stools, thirst with desire to drink, flushed face, fever, irritability, foul breath, fullness and distention of the chest, hypochondria and abdomen, poor appetite, dark urine. Red tongue with thin coating, dim purple superficial venule of the index finger.

Treatment principle   Clear Heat, moisten the Large Intestine and remove stagnation.

Prescription   Clearing Large Intestine Channel (see Fig. 5-75), clearing Stomach Channel (see Fig. 5-76),

165

clearing Spleen Channel (see Fig. 5-77), pushing Banmen (see Fig. 5-78), kneading Guiwei (see Fig. 5-79) and pushing down Qijiegu (see Fig. 5-80).
Medium   Talcum or sesame oil.

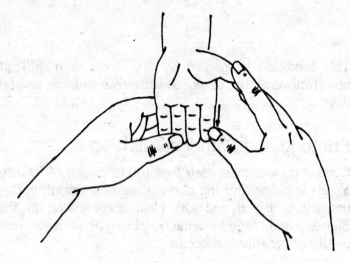

Fig. 5-75   Clearing Large Intestine Channel

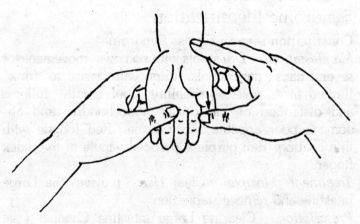

Fig. 5-76   Clearing Stomach Channel

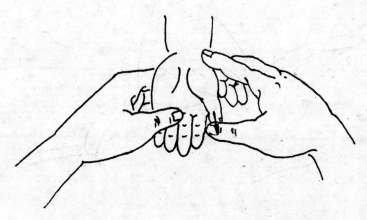

Fig. 5-77   Clearing Spleen Channel

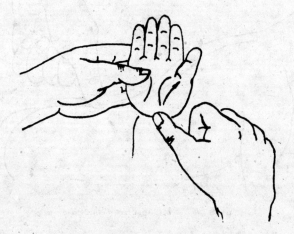

Fig. 5-78   Pushing Banmen

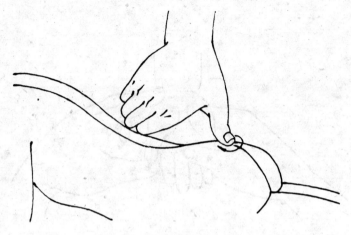

Fig. 5-79 Kneading Guiwei

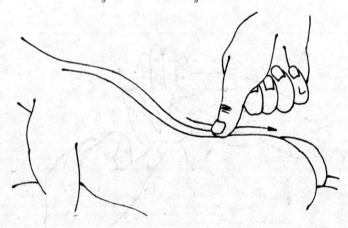

Fig. 5-80 Pushing down Qijiegu

Constipation seen in Deficiency Syndrome

Manifestations Pale face without luster, listlessness, emaciation, crying with low thin voice, difficult bowel movement, pale lips. Pale tongue with thin coating, dim pale superficial venule of the index finger.

Treatment principle Reinforce the Kidney and pro-

168

mote Kidney Qi; nourish Blood and moisten the Large Intestine.

Prescription   Reinforcing Spleen Channel (see Fig. 5-81), pushing Sanguan (see Fig. 5-82), circular rubbing Shenque (REN 8) (see Fig. 5-83), pushing down Qijiegu (see Fig. 5-84) and kneading Zusanli (ST 36) (see Fig. 5-85).

Medium   Talcum.

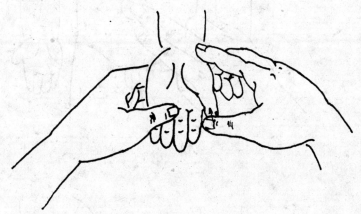

Fig. 5-81   Reinforcing Spleen Channel

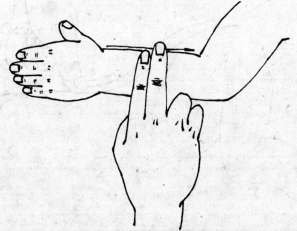

Fig. 5-82   Pushing Sanguan

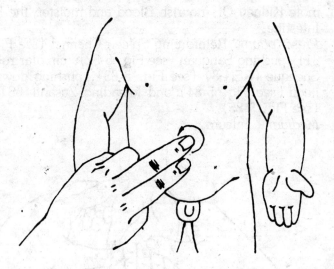

Fig. 5-83   Circular rubbing Shenque

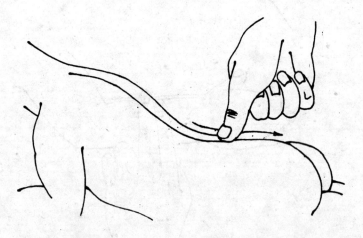

Fig. 5-84   Pushing down Qijiegu

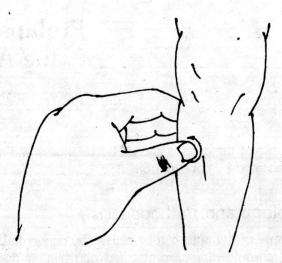

Fig. 5-85   Kneading Zusanli

Prolapse of the Anus

Prolapse of the anus is caused by weakness and may be complicated by constipation.

Etiology and Pathogenesis

Prolapse of the anus can be caused by congenital weakness, chronic illness, protracted diarrhea or dysentery leading to Deficiency of Spleen and Lung Qi, and finally sinking of Qi occurs. It can also be brought about by Damp Heat retained in the Middle Jiao leading to stagnation of Qi and dry stools.

Treatment Based on Syndrome Identification

Prolapse of the anus due to Sinking of Middle Qi
Manifestations   Emaciation, dusky complexion, listlessness, spontaneous sweating, no desire to speak, prolapse of the anus during bowel movement, no redness and pain of the anus. Pale tongue with thin white coating, pale superficial venule of the index finger.
Treatment principle   Reinforce the Middle Jiao and tonify Qi; promote Qi and lift the anus.
Prescription   Reinforcing Spleen Channel (see Fig. 5-86), reinforcing Lung Channel (see Fig. 5-87), rein-

forcing Large Intestine Channel (see Fig. 5-88), pushing Sanguan (see Fig. 5-89), kneading Baihui (DU 20) (see Fig. 5-90), pushing up Qijiegu (see Fig. 5-91), kneading Guiwei (see Fig. 5-92) and kneading Zusanli (ST 36) (see Fig. 5-93).

Medium   Talcum.

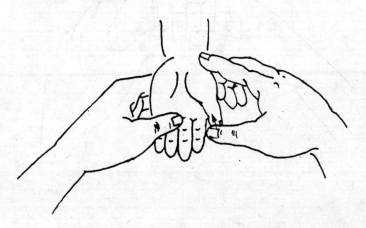

Fig. 5-86   Reinforcing Spleen Channel

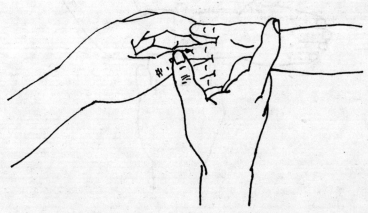

Fig. 5-87   Reinforcing Lung Channel

173

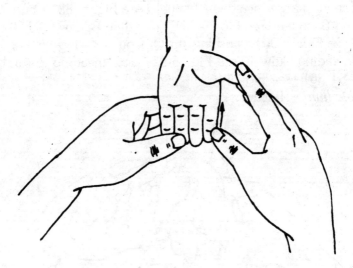

Fig. 5-88   Reinforcing Large Intestine Channel

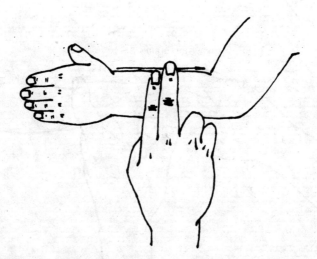

Fig. 5-89   Pushing Sanguan

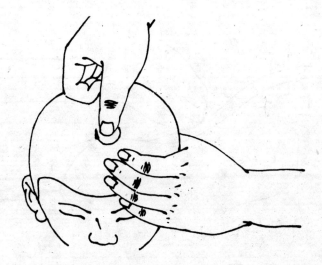

Fig. 5-90   Kneading Baihui

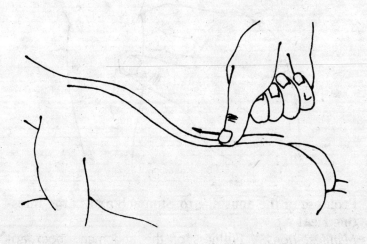

Fig. 5-91   Pushing up Qijiegu

175

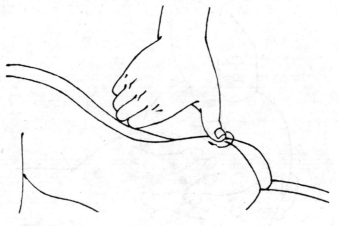

Fig. 5-92   Kneading Guiwei

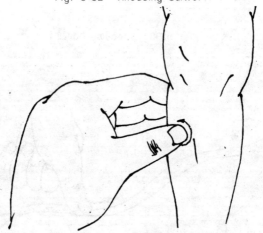

Fig. 5-93   Kneading Zusanli

Prolapse of the anus due to Stomach and Large Intestine Heat

Manifestations   Fullness of the abdomen, poor appetite, restlessness, hot feeling in the abdomen at night, dry stool or loose stools with sticky discharge, redness and swelling around the anus. Red tongue with

176

thin yellow coating, dark purple superficial venule of the index finger.

Treatment principle   Clear Heat and remove Damp; benefit the Large Intestine and improve the prolapse.

Prescription   Clearing and reinforcing Spleen Channel (see Fig. 5-94), clearing Stomach Channel (see Fig. 5-95), clearing Large Intestine Channel (see Fig. 5-96), kneading Guiwei (see Fig. 5-97) and pushing down Qijiegu (see Fig. 5-98).

Medium   Talcum or cold water.

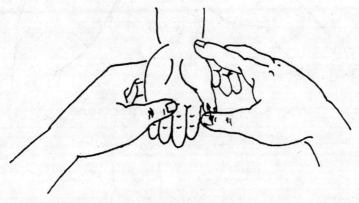

Fig. 5-94   Clearing and reinforcing Spleen Channel

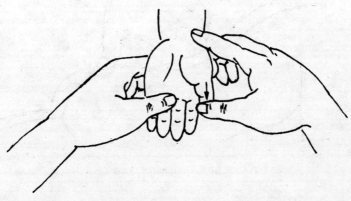

Fig. 5-95   Clearing Stomach Channel

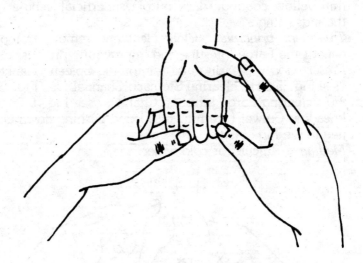

Fig. 5-96 Clearing Large Intestine Channel

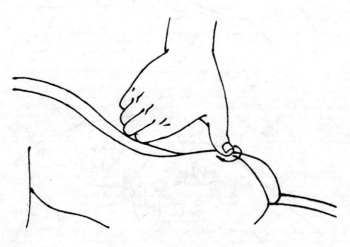

Fig. 5-97 Kneading Guiwei

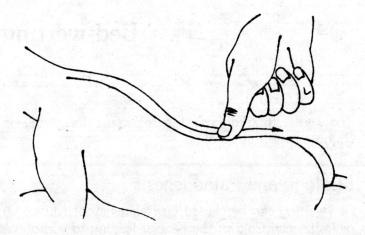

Fig. 5-98   Pushing down Qijiegu

Bed-wetting

The bed-wetting discussed here occurs frequently in children over 3 years old.

Etiology and Pathogenesis

Bed-wetting can be caused by Deficiency of Kidney Qi or Deficiency Cold of the Kidney leading to consolidation of urine. It can also be brought about by the downward flow of Damp Heat leading to dysfunction of the Bladder.

Treatment Based on Syndrome Identification

Bed-wetting seen in Deficiency Cold Syndrome

Manifestations   Pale face, weak mentality, soreness and weakness of the lumbar area and knees, cold limbs, poor appetite, irritability, drowsiness. Pale tongue with thin white coating, red and floating superficial venule of the index finger.

Treatment principle   Warm the Kidney and reinforce the Spleen; tonify Qi and consolidate the Bladder.

Prescription   Reinforcing Spleen Channel (see Fig. 5-99), reinforcing Kidney Channel (see Fig. 5-100), pushing Sanguan (see Fig. 5-101), kneading Erma (see Fig. 5-102), kneading Pishu (BL 20) (see Fig. 5-103), kneading Feishu (BL 13) (see Fig. 5-104), kneading

Shenshu (BL 23) (see Fig. 5-105), circular rubbing
Shenque (REN 8) (see Fig. 5-106) and circular rubbing
Guanyuan (REN 4) (see Fig. 5-107).
Medium Talcum.

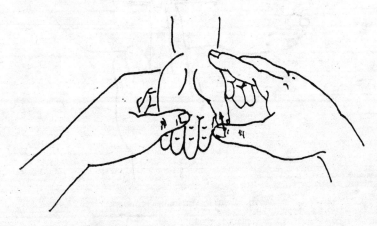

Fig. 5-99   Reinforcing Spleen Channel

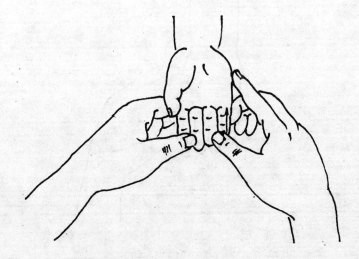

Fig. 5-100   Reinforcing Kidney Channel

181

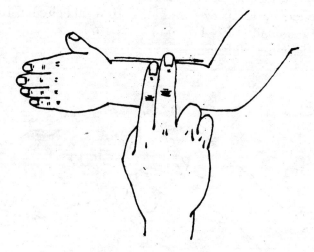

Fig. 5-101   Pushing Sanguan

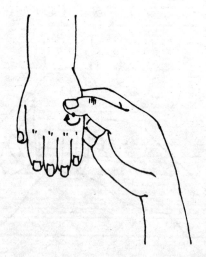

Fig. 5-102   Kneading Erma

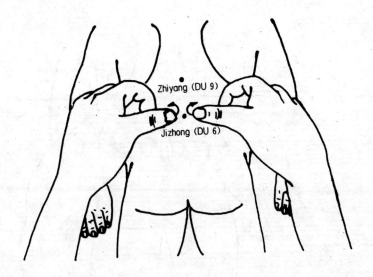

Fig. 5-103   Kneading Pishu

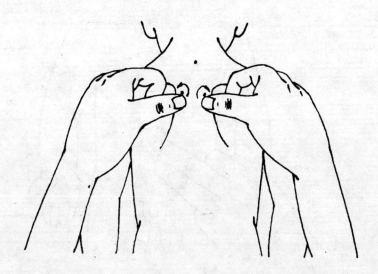

Fig. 5-104   Kneading Feishu

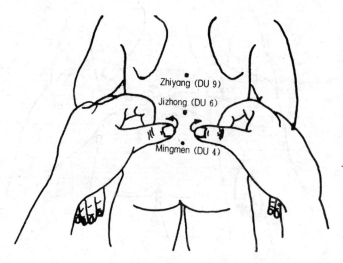

Fig. 5-105   Kneading Shenshu

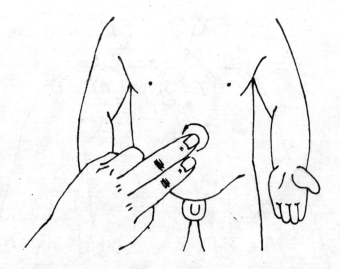

Fig. 5-106   Circular rubbing Shenque

184

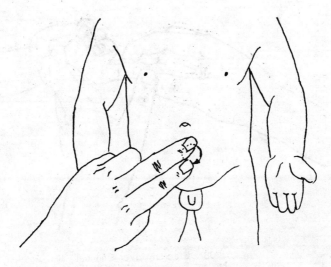

Fig. 5-107   Circular rubbing Guanyuan

Bed-wetting seen in Excess Syndrome

Manifestations   Flushed face, red lips, irritability, thirst with desire for cold drinks, restlessness, five palm heat, frequent urgent urination, bed-wetting with yellow foul urine. Red tongue with thin yellow coating, dark red superficial venule of the index finger.

Treatment principle   Purge Liver and clear Heat; regulate the flow of Qi and consolidate the Bladder.

Prescription   Clearing Liver Channel (see Fig. 5-108), clearing Heart Channel (see Fig. 5-109), clearing Small Intestine Channel (see Fig. 5-110), pushing up the Galaxy (see Fig. 5-111), kneading Xinshu (BL 15) (see Fig. 5-112), kneading Ganshu (BL 18) (see Fig. 5-113), kneading Danshu (BL 19) (see Fig. 5-114) and kneading Shenshu (BL 23) (see Fig. 5-115).

Medium   Talcum or cold water.

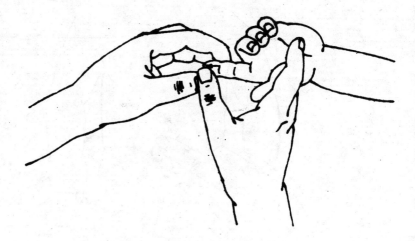

Fig. 5-108   Clearing Liver Channel

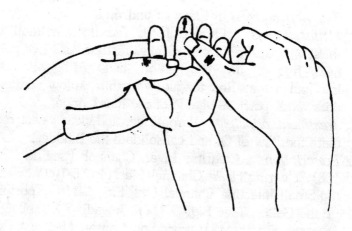

Fig. 5-109   Clearing Heart Channel

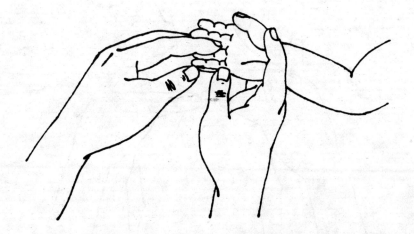

Fig. 5-110   Clearing Small Intestine Channel

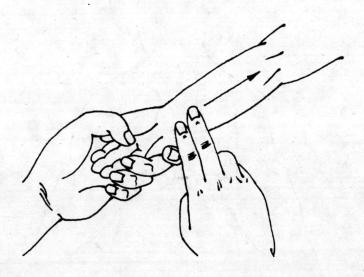

Fig. 5-111   Pushing up the Galaxy

187

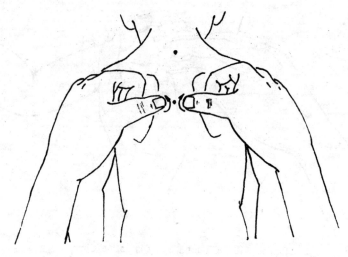

Fig. 5-112   Kneading Xinshu

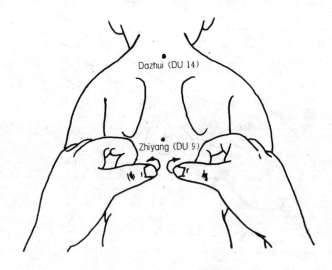

Fig. 5-113   Kneading Ganshu

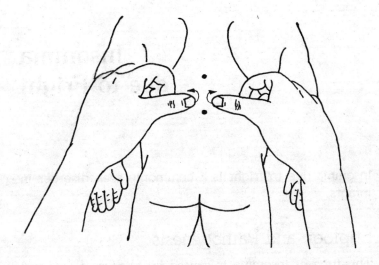

Fig. 5-114 Kneading Danshu

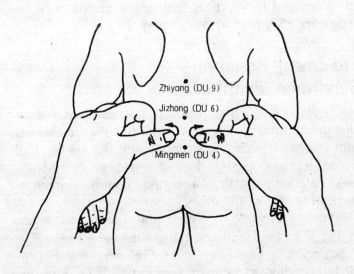

Zhiyang (DU 9)

Jizhong (DU 6)

Mingmen (DU 4)

Fig. 5-115 Kneading Shenshu

Insomnia
due to Fright

Insomnia due to fright is a commonly seen disorder in infants.

Etiology and Pathogenesis

This type of insomnia is caused by attacks of fear and terror leading to dysfunction of the Heart in storing vitality and mentality. Fear may cause disorders of Qi, and terror may lead to descending of Qi.

Treatment Based on Syndrome Identification

Manifestations Weakness, listlessness, pale face, blue-green around the nose and mouth, restlessness with spasm of limbs, or sleeping with the eyelids half-closed, chronic crying, loss of appetite, or bed-wetting. Pale tongue with thin coating, light blue-green superficial venule of the index finger.

Treatment principle Check the Liver and relieve fright; calm the Heart and tranquilize the Mind.

Prescription Checking Liver Channel (see Fig. 5-116), kneading Xiaotianxin (see Fig. 5-117), kneading Erma (see Fig. 5-118), pushing Xinmen (see Fig. 5-119), reinforcing Kidney Channel (see Fig. 5-120) and

marking and kneading Wuzhijie (see Fig. 5-121).
Medium Talcum.

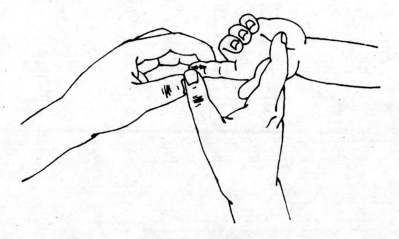

Fig. 5-116   Checking Liver Channel

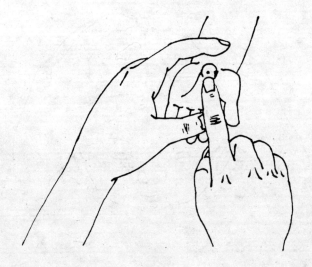

Fig. 5-117   Kneading Xiaotianxin

191

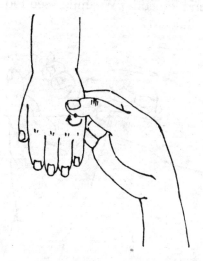

Fig. 5-118   Kneading Erma

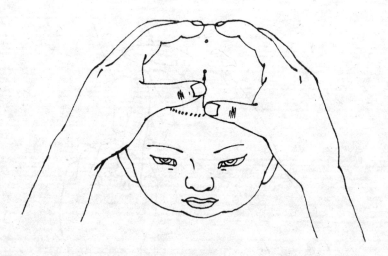

Fig. 5-119   Pushing Xinmen

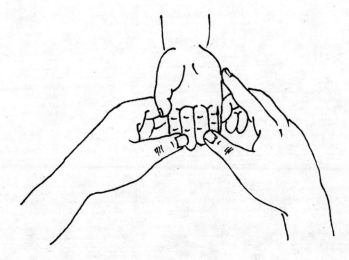

Fig. 5-120　Reinforcing Kidney Channel

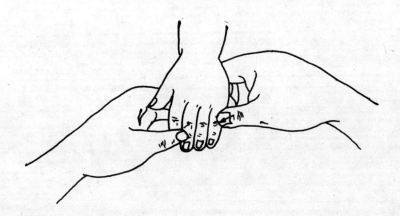

Fig. 5-121　Marking and kneading Wuzhijie

193

ATTACHED
FINGERS

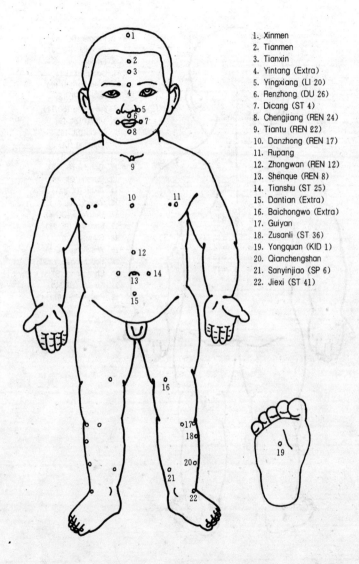

1. Xinmen
2. Tianmen
3. Tianxin
4. Yintang (Extra)
5. Yingxiang (LI 20)
6. Renzhong (DU 26)
7. Dicang (ST 4)
8. Chengjiang (REN 24)
9. Tiantu (REN 22)
10. Danzhong (REN 17)
11. Rupang
12. Zhongwan (REN 12)
13. Shenque (REN 8)
14. Tianshu (ST 25)
15. Dantian (Extra)
16. Baichongwo (Extra)
17. Guiyan
18. Zusanli (ST 36)
19. Yongquan (KID 1)
20. Qianchengshan
21. Sanyinjiao (SP 6)
22. Jiexi (ST 41)

Fig. 1 Commonly used points on the front of the torso

197

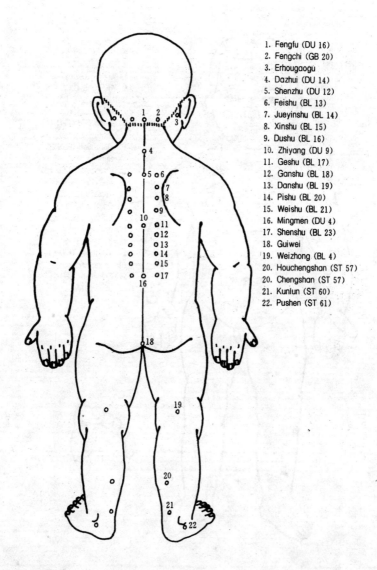

1. Fengfu (DU 16)
2. Fengchi (GB 20)
3. Erhougaogu
4. Dazhui (DU 14)
5. Shenzhu (DU 12)
6. Feishu (BL 13)
7. Jueyinshu (BL 14)
8. Xinshu (BL 15)
9. Dushu (BL 16)
10. Zhiyang (DU 9)
11. Geshu (BL 17)
12. Ganshu (BL 18)
13. Danshu (BL 19)
14. Pishu (BL 20)
15. Weishu (BL 21)
16. Mingmen (DU 4)
17. Shenshu (BL 23)
18. Guiwei
19. Weizhong (BL 4)
20. Houchengshan (ST 57)
20. Chengshan (ST 57)
21. Kunlun (ST 60)
22. Pushen (ST 61)

Fig. 2 Commonly used points on the back of the torso

198

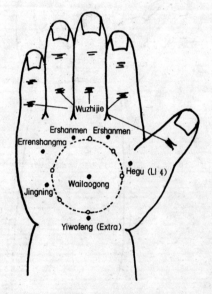

Fig. 3 Commonly used points on the
dorsum of the hand

199

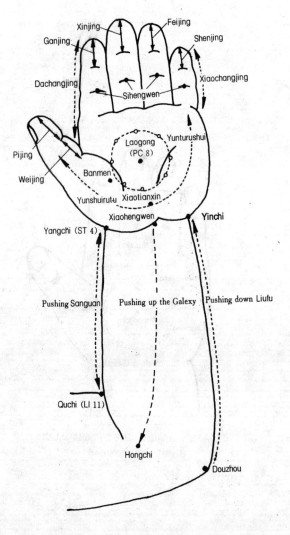

Fig. 4 Commonly used points on the
palm and forearm.

200

婴幼儿保健按摩图解

主　　编　曲敬喜　王庆林
副 主 编　王焕国　刘日和
　　　　　高连军
翻　　译　陈平
绘　　图　刘辉宇　郭磊
英文编辑　马莎·维奇(美)
责任编辑　李　宇　仲彭军

*

山东科学技术出版社出版
中国济南市玉函路 16 号　邮政编码 250002
中国济南新华印刷厂印刷
中国国际图书贸易总公司发行
中国北京车公庄西路 35 号
北京邮政信箱第 399 号　邮政编码 100044

*

1997 年(大 32 开)　1 版 1 次
ISBN 7 - 5331 - 2049 - 3
R·598
08200
14 - E - 3030P